MW00466697

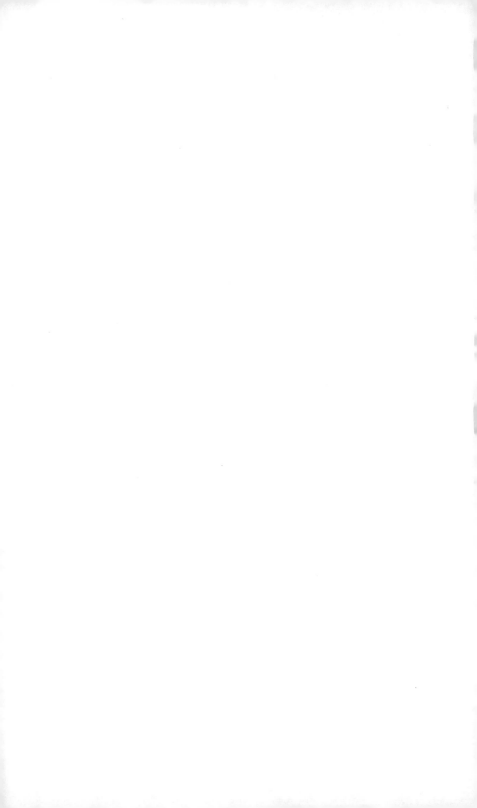

IT WAS
ONLY A
MOMENT
AGO

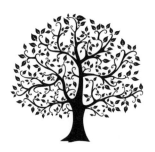

More Stories of Healing and Wisdom
Along Life's Journey

IT WAS ONLY A MOMENT AGO

More Stories of Healing and Wisdom
Along Life's Journey

WILLIAM E. HABLITZEL, MD

SUNSHINE RIDGE PUBLISHING

It Was Only A Moment Ago: More Stories of Healing and Wisdom Along Life's Journey/ by William E. Hablitzel, MD

Copyright ©2011 Hablitzel, William E.

Published in the United States by Sunshine Ridge Publishing

Sunshine Ridge Publishing
P.O. Box 69
Blue Creek, Ohio 45616

Publisher's Cataloging-In-Publication Data
Hablitzel, William E.
It was only a moment ago : more stories of healing and wisdom along life's journey / William E. Hablitzel. -- 1st ed.
p. ; cm.
ISBN: 978-0-9772185-4-7
1. Physician and patient--Anecdotes. 2. Medicine--Anecdotes. 3. Conduct of life.
I. Title.
R705 .H33 2010
610.696   2010926460

Printed in the United States of America

Book Design by Brion Sausser (www.bookcreatives.com)

To Charlie and Ellen, who shared with me life
that I might otherwise know little of.
To John Harricharan, in whose spark I discovered the written word.
And to my mother, for starting me on the most extraordinary journey.

Contents

Foreword

For those in the healing profession or in need of healing, *It Was Only a Moment Ago*, by master story teller, physician, and teacher, Bill Hablitzel, demonstrates that the power to heal resides in all of us. With elegant words, exquisite prose, and a deep sense of what is essential for restoring well-being, Bill Hablitzel illuminates healing as an experience which must include the soul as well as the body.

Written in a beautiful and gentle style, Bill Hablitzel invites you into his life, sharing with you those who have been his teachers of the healing process. Few doctors are as honest as Bill in acknowledging that the wisdom they gain from their patients often exceeds what they learn in their medical training; few doctors recognize what true healing is and few have discovered what Bill has—the healing power of love, touch, a change of perspective, compassion, and living in the Now.

Be prepared to be touched, inspired, deeply moved, and informed about how you, too, can create your own miracles of healing. Bill Hablitzel tenderly and lovingly intertwines stories of teachers from his childhood with those of his patients, students, and colleagues who are now his teachers, weaving a fabric that warms your heart and moves you to be open to possibilities that you are not only touched by the extraordinary but that you are extraordinary.

Additionally, Bill's teachers, amazing role models and courageous souls who have learned to meet their challenges with hope, love, and joy, will forever change your perspective about what healing is. They will remain with you forever, as though you had read about them *Only a Moment Ago.*

Awaiting you in the pages that follow is a powerful, inspirational, and heartwarming collection of stories filled with exquisite, yet tender and comforting wisdom for all of us who view life as a magnificent journey of blossoming into our potential and living our dreams. This is highly recommended reading for everyone in the healing profession, as well as those seeking their own healing, feel-good experience.

Susan Barbara Apollon
Intuitive psychologist and author of
Touched by the Extraordinary
www.TouchedByTheExtraordinary.com

Introduction

L ife can change in the blink of an eye. With the wrench of a steering wheel, that college final, the wedding rehearsal, or the promotion at work becomes instantly irrelevant. With a pain in the chest, the dreams of retirement evaporate. In the succinct words of a diagnosis, that argument with the kids, those unpaid bills, or the neighbor's unkempt lawn become so trivial. With the rumble of the earth, a wall of water, or winds from the sea, entire nations can simply disappear.

Why do bad things have to happen? It was a question once asked of me by a medical student who struggled with the darkness he hadn't expected to find in medicine, although I suspect it is a question most of us have asked ourselves a time or two. Indeed, there is darkness and we invite it into our lives.

It comes in the newspaper headlines of scandal and politics that we find on our doorstep every morning. It comes in the narrative of fear and blame that we hear on the radio as we drive to work. It comes in the images of atrocities inflicted in the name of religion that play repeatedly on our television monitors. It comes in the lyrics of our music, the video games we play, and in the drama of the movies we watch.

Darkness is a powerful energy. It soaks deep into our souls and changes us. It makes us ill. It fills doctors' offices and emergency rooms with pain, fatigue, anxiety, and all manner of unhappiness.

They come seeking cure, but cure just isn't enough.

When I completed medical school and residency, I was exceptionally well trained. I could halt a raging infection, temper out-of-control blood pressure, or even restart a silent heart, but I knew little of the darkness that inflicted my patients' lives. While I knew all about curing, I knew nothing of healing, and the realization that there was a profound difference between the two took me by surprise. Perhaps an even bigger surprise was that my greatest teachers of healing did not come from the lecture hall, the authors of journal articles, or medical grand rounds. My greatest teachers were the patients that I cared for.

People will tell their physicians things that they wouldn't dream of telling family or their closest of friends. Combine that willingness to share with the circumstances in which people seek out their physicians—illness, injury, stress, profound life challenge, and yes, even death—and physicians are privileged to see life stripped down to its nuts and bolts; to its very essence. Amidst that essence can be found incredible wisdom and secrets to a life filled with meaning, abundance, and uncommon happiness.

You don't have to become ill, suffer injury, develop cancer, or even face death in order to experience the wisdom and discover the life-changing secrets that can be found in such situations, we can learn from those that have been there.

We come into this world filled with endless happiness, unbounded peace, and seeds carried from another place that have the potential to grow into incredible wisdom. All too quickly, we grasp the expectations of others, surrender our gifts of youth, and invite darkness into our lives. Perhaps healing is the journey that we once again take to find that peace. It is a journey with many twists and turns, but there are many teachers along the way to keep us centered upon our path.

I invite you to spend part of your journey with the special teachers found within the pages that follow. Although their names and circumstances have been changed to preserve privacy, their stories are real. They are stories that come from the depths of the human soul and bubble to the surface as extraordinary wisdom. They are stories that will fill you with wonder, hope, and the awareness that we are not alone. They are stories that will heal your life. Inside you will find laughter, excitement, and even tears. Some of the tears may very well be your own.

Our journey here is a brief one. It only lasts a lifetime.

William E. Hablitzel, MD

CHAPTER 1

You Find What You Look For

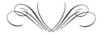

Happiness is a butterfly, which, when pursued, is always just beyond
your grasp, but which, if you will sit down quietly, may alight upon you.

NATHANIEL HAWTHORNE

The clearest way into the universe is through a forest wilderness.

JOHN MUIR

It doesn't seem that long ago when the ways of the fire service held captive my dreams of success and meaning. It seems just the other day that as a young man, I was confident that the years of study that awaited me in medical school would lead to great satisfaction and happiness. When I joined the faculty-practice at the medical school, I felt certain the path would take me to all that I was looking for in life. Now decades later, those things have led me here. It is a place that many would find curious for a physician, but there is no place I would rather be.

The large flat rock upon which I sit is uncommonly comfortable, but it always has been. In the heat of summer, it provides a refreshing coolness, while on the coldest winter days it radiates warmth from the depths of the earth below. Its texture has softness to it, as if it was sculpted through the millennia solely for the comfort of man. I often find myself wondering how many others before me have sat in this spot.

Nestled between two ridges among the rugged hills of southern Ohio is a place of great beauty—beauty of such depth one can become lost within it. The small stream that wanders across the valley floor explores every stone and fallen branch as it twists and turns with childlike glee before slipping away into the wooded distance. The hardwood forest pauses here and gradually opens to a pristine clearing reminiscent of the sanctuary offered by a great cathedral, its towering walls and arched ceilings moving rhythmically in the gentle breeze. It is a sacred place.

It is called Demazie Hollow, but nobody seems to know why. Perhaps its name comes from the days when the Shawnee roamed and hunted these woods. Perhaps they too were drawn to this very rock and would sit and marvel at the beauty that surrounded them. In the stillness, you could almost feel their presence and the wisdom they left behind.

A tufted titmouse led me to this place, not long after I joined the faculty practice at the teaching hospital. A card from Betts Unger had reminded me of earlier days when we walked the marshes and fields of northern Ohio in search of birds. It had been many years since I had been birding and I longed once again to feel the peace that nature had once brought to me. It was peace that eluded me on morning rounds at the Teaching Hospital, peace that hid somewhere among the endless stream of patients that filled my schedule each day, and peace that couldn't be found within the pages of medical journals that sat upon my desk.

That old pair of binoculars fit in my grasp like the hand of an old friend. The worn and aging bird book in my pocket was filled with countless notes of discovery, many penned by the hand of a boy. Standing alongside that wooded road, there was a strong sense of déjà vu—I had felt this excitement before. The call of the tufted titmouse from a nearby redbud brought a smile to my face—it was the first bird that Betts had taught me about. Strange that it would be the first bird to greet me here.

I followed that titmouse down a narrow and poorly worn path, no doubt a trail forged across the forest floor by passing deer. With my every approach, it would move farther into the woods and pause invitingly, as if leading me to a special place. The path melted into the opening of a large clearing, the entrance guarded by the largest oak tree I had ever seen. It was a red oak with a crown that towered high above those of its neighbors. Wild blackberry with long arching canes laden with fruit, rhododendron, multifora rose, and wildflowers—an abundance of wildflowers—painted a magical setting. Nearby was the large rock upon which I now sit. It has been a place of rest, of contemplation, of wonder, and of understanding. It seems a strange place for a physician to have discovered healing.

In medical school, we are taught all about cure. Countless hours spent over a cadaver in the gross anatomy laboratory, peering into the secrets of human tissue through a microscope, or mastering the intricacies of biochemical pathways to help us define what is normal so that we might come to recognize disease. Hospital rounds, thick medical journals, and endless lectures instruct how to cure that disease. It can be a sobering realization for a young doctor that cure just may not be enough.

The Teaching Hospital can be a magical place. Those in need are drawn here. The latest that science has to offer becomes routine. The best of technology is unleashed here. The brightest of our profession practice here and through their excellence we all become better. The satisfaction of making a difficult diagnosis is dwarfed by the fulfillment experienced in watching an ill patient improve through your efforts. Among the magic that happens here is the transition from student to physician, a metamorphosis that few are privileged to watch, and fewer still come to share.

Not long ago, I sat in the nursing station on the medical floor of the Teaching Hospital. It is one of the busiest floors in the hospital and chaos is typically the rule rather than the exception. But it is a controlled chaos, one that fosters dozens of new patient admissions and discharges every day. It is a large area that supports some forty patient rooms, but it is always uncomfortably crowded. Nurses, students, physicians, social workers and therapists all compete for the same space in which to do their work. Every flat surface is a precious commodity and it's not unusual to see patient charts balanced on top of computer monitors and copiers as clinicians frantically attempt to document their daily work.

If there is peace to be found in the hospital, it will not be encountered here. A sense of urgency hangs in the air like a fog. Everything is in motion—harried movement that echoes the scarcity of time. Conversation flows from every corner of the room and with the ringing of telephones, impatient pagers, and the beeping of monitors, it creates a raucous brew. But on this day, the nursing station was particularly lacking in peace.

It was the first day of July, the day when a new class of medical school graduates started their careers as doctors in hospitals all across the country. It was the day when observers became participants. As demanding as medical school can be, there is security, if not solace, in the realization that as students they can do little harm. But on this day, reality would change. With the turn of a page on the calendar, their signature suddenly carried the weight of a physician's order, and with it the heavy burden of responsibility.

One day was much like the next at the Teaching Hospital. Urgency and crises were so commonplace that they became routine. Critical laboratory results, patients in respiratory distress, piercing alarms from cardiac monitors, and the myriad other insults to equanimity hardly raised an eyebrow or quickened a pulse among those who made the hospital home. Nothing seemed to trouble them or challenge their practiced composure, except for the early days of July.

July touched everyone at the Teaching Hospital. Nurses watched over their kingdom with atypical angst, scrutinizing every order and pondering the accuracy of every decision made. Unit clerks struggled to explain hospital policies to newcomers, policies that more often than not defied explanation. Medical residents discovered that it was much easier to care for a patient than it was to watch a new colleague learn how to provide that care. Faculty physicians hovered nervously about and always seemed to be in the way. Therapists, transporters, students, and all the rest worked with imposing silence, silence more typical of a funeral home than a busy hospital. Even the patients sensed something special as incredibly young-looking eyes peered at them during morning rounds—the brand new interns had started.

The energy of those days touched no one more profoundly than the young interns. There is no other time on the journey to become a physician when doubt is greater, when the future seems more uncertain, and when fear's grasp is stronger. So powerful is the experience that the memories will survive a lifetime. The new doctors were easy to spot in the nursing station. Clad in pristine white coats, pockets bulging with notes, reference books, and electronics, they would jump in unison with the sound of every pager and grope at pockets and belts to see if it was their pager that was calling them to action. It was a strange sight to witness—almost like a collective seizure.

One young doctor in particular caught my eye. She was young, seemingly too young to be a physician, and I smiled at the realization that with each passing year, the interns and students seemed to get younger to me. She sat across the table from me as I wrote a progress note on one of my patients that had been hospitalized the night before. A patient's chart sat open before her and she stared at it anxiously as if it contained a heavy burden. Periodically, she would dig through her pockets as if looking for lost car keys, or frantically thumb through the pages of a reference book that she extracted from her white coat. In a room full of people, she seemed so alone.

Her restlessness made it difficult for me to concentrate on my work and after the better part of ten minutes watching, I simply couldn't take it anymore.

"Excuse me," I said softly. "Is there something that I can do to help?"

You would have thought I had shot her with a gun. Startled, she sat bolt upright. Her face reflected a mixture of both surprise and embarrassment.

"No," she said in a hushed voice, "I'm fine."

I looked into those eyes that peered at me from beneath neatly trimmed bangs. They were kind but frightened-appearing eyes and in the corner of one of them I was almost certain I could see a tear.

"Are you sure?" I asked again. "I'm pretty good at solving problems."

She sat in silence for a few moments as if troubled that asking for help might be seen as a sign of weakness.

"It's these orders," she finally said in surrender. "I don't know how to write *aspirin.*"

"I'm sorry?" I said. The question seemed too simple, even for July 1st.

"He's a cardiac patient," she stammered, "and I'm supposed to put him on aspirin. I don't know how to write *aspirin.*"

Stifling a smile and with the most serious face I could muster, I looked her in the eyes and said, "I usually start with the letter *a.*"

She just stared at me, much like a deer in headlights. All emotion had drained from her face, including the fear that I had seen just moments earlier. It was a full minute before I detected the faint trace of a smile. Slowly it grew. It was as infectious as the organisms that we treat and soon we both smiled broadly at each other.

"I thought you were serious!" she exclaimed with a sigh of relief.

I glanced at the ID badge that hung from the breast pocket of her coat. Beneath her picture was inscribed, 'Samantha Smyth, M.D.' "So, Doctor Smyth," I asked, "how is your first day going?"

She jumped a little at hearing her name, or perhaps at the title of Doctor. "No, no," she said quickly, "it's Samantha. But my friends call me Sam."

Her smile softened visibly. "Strange," she noted wistfully, "I always wanted to be called Doctor. Now I don't want anyone to know."

"So, Samantha," I gently prodded, "how is your first day going?"

Her smile slowly faded into the turmoil that surrounded us and fear once again crept into those eyes. "I'm not sure that I know," she said softly. "All through medical school I looked forward to this day—it got me through many tough times. I thought I had found what I was looking for, but this is not what I was expecting."

"You are going to do just fine," I reassured her. "You wouldn't be sitting here if the department didn't have confidence in your ability. It won't be long until you have confidence in them too."

"I wish I could believe that," she said ruefully.

"You can," I said emphatically, "because I've been there. All doctors have. It's part of our journey. Let me tell you a secret about the attending physician on your team. I can remember when he sat in this room on his first day. He wanted to quit before lunch. He spent half the day in the bathroom."

"What happened?" she asked in a hushed voice, her eyes growing wide.

"He became a fine physician," I said. "There are two things that you need to remember: First, you are never alone. There will always be someone around to help you—residents, attending physicians, and even the nurses. And you know what? Even your patients will help you to help them. All you have to do is ask the right questions and then take the time to listen for the answers. It's something that takes many of us a long time to learn. Some docs never figure it out."

If she didn't appear convinced, at least she seemed relieved by what I told her. "And what's the second thing?" she asked.

"That we find what we look for," I said, "even when we do not realize what we are looking for."

A gentle but persistent tapping guided my thoughts back to the clearing in Demazie Hollow. A downy woodpecker was working on the side of the red oak, very intent on discovering what secrets might be found beneath a sliver of loosened bark. As it probed and pried, those words consumed my thoughts—we find what we look for.

Betts Unger used those words the first time I walked with her in search of birds. George walked with us. Neither ever having married, brother and sister lived together and taught English at my hometown high school. During the week, they would teach grammar, sentence structure, and the love of literature. Weekends would find them together savoring the beauty and wisdom they found in nature. What once seemed an amazing coincidence that our paths would cross one day in a deserted hallway after school, I now know had been much more. There are no coincidences.

Throughout high school and much of college, weekends were spent with the Ungers. Spring and summer vacations brought travel to distant lands for exploration, adventure, and always for birds. Separated in age by some five decades, we appeared to others as grandson and grandparents, an illusion I believe they treasured. But we were more than family—we were friends.

Our weekly journey often took us down a wooded path of a wildlife sanctuary, as it was always profitable for birds. Not far from the start of the trail was a bench that overlooked a small pond. One morning we came upon an elderly man sitting on the bench. He was frail and seemed strangely out of place. A walker stood next to him. Oxygen tubing ran from his nose to a green cylinder that hung from his shoulder. The binoculars he held in his hands shook visibly and I wondered how he could see anything through them. As we passed, Betts's greeting brought a smile to his face.

"Do you know that man?" I asked.

"No," she said, "but I know many others like him."

She smiled at my quizzical look and asked, "What better place to come with a problem?"

Every week, we would see that old man sitting on the bench. Perhaps we had simply grown accustomed to him, but I was rather certain that his binoculars didn't shake as much after a month or two. As the spring migration flowed into the nesting season, a cane leaned against the bench where his walker once stood. By the time fall migration started, the oxygen cylinder was gone and by Thanksgiving, so was the cane.

One day, with winter's first snow still clinging to the trees, the bench sat conspicuously empty. A short walk farther down the trail stood a man peering intently into a tangle of wild grape with binoculars. We too stood and studied the twisted vines that swayed gently in the crisp breeze. From its midst emerged a tufted titmouse, its crest rising and falling as if in greeting. With a smile, the man lowered the glasses from his eyes and turned to us. I stared in disbelief at the once frail man who no longer sat on the bench. He bowed subtly, almost reverently, and silently moved off down the trail.

We never spoke of that old man—words simply could not add to the moment—but when I would sit on that bench with Betts, she always took notice of the powerful stillness that could be found there, stillness that could change us. While it would be many years before medical school professors would teach me about cure, Betts had already planted the seeds of understanding about healing. Those seeds sprouted here in Demazie Hollow, their growth nourished by the paradox that is this place.

The peace I couldn't find on morning rounds or in the office was always waiting for me here, and once found, it would accompany me to the hospital every day. On those days, I found more than medicine—I found what I was looking for.

CHAPTER 2

The Epiphany of More

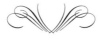

*No man can reveal to you nothing but that which already
lies half-asleep in the dawning of your knowledge.*

KAHLIL GIBRAN

*There are some things which cannot be learned quickly, and time,
which is all we have, must be paid heavily for their acquiring.
They are the very simplest things and because it takes a man's
life to know them, the little new that each man gets from life
is very costly and the only heritage he has to leave.*

JOHN MUIR

It seems such a simple thing—the awareness that there is more to
our existence than that which we can see, touch, experience, or
even understand—but it is the energy that fuels profound evolution,
no less than the discovery of fire or the realization that our flat world
was not the center of the universe. Sometimes, the awareness strikes
us all at once. More often than not, it speaks with a gentle voice, one
so soft and unobtrusive that it rests unnoticed deep within our soul
until it is warmed and nourished enough to germinate into a thought

that haunts our days until we act upon it. And so it has been along my journey.

We interpret our world through the experiences of youth, the values of our fathers, and the expectations of others. We believe as we have been taught. After years of college, medical school, and residency, physicians find their truths imbedded deeply within the scientific method, medical literature, and technology. Mentors perpetuate tradition, and with it a hubris that narrows vision and closes the mind to the richness of unconsidered possibilities. When the student is ready, the ancient Buddhist proverb tells us, the teacher will appear. The truly special teachers often appear before we are ready, their lessons so important that they wait patiently in our thoughts until we are prepared to listen.

While not aware of them at the time, these teachers started appearing the instant I touched the lives of others. Long before I started medical school, I could hear their whispers. One warm spring night, the whisper brought a shiver down my spine.

I had been a paramedic for only a few days when the shrill tone came across the radio alerting the fire station of an emergency call. My work on the ambulance as a volunteer inspired me more than any college course ever had, inspiration that overwhelmed the plans of a premed student on an uncertain journey. Without a moment's hesitation, I took a quarter off from school to seize the rare opportunity to be trained as a paramedic. As I sat in the ambulance waiting for the rest of my team to arrive, I struggled with the burden that had consumed my thoughts all day long—do I return to school or accept the just-offered full-time job as one of our community's first paramedics?

The transmission over the radio redirected my thoughts to the more urgent matters at hand. The first police units signaled that they were at the scene. It was a 10-31, a motor vehicle accident. It didn't take many moments for the officer's voice to return. I knew him and liked him. The stress in his voice made me anxious.

"Unit 12 to headquarters," the pressured voice said, "advise Medic-One that this is a 10-99. We have trapped victims. You had better roll the fire department as well."

No sooner had the radio grown quiet when the fire station's bell rang. Even though I sat in the ambulance, its motor idling on the front apron of the station, I still jumped at the sound of the bell. It was an evil thing that seemed capable of reaching deep into your soul with icy cold fingers. I would never get accustomed to it.

I always felt a quickened pulse when I pulled the ambulance out into traffic, but this night I could not deny the apprehension that I struggled to keep secret from my colleagues. I had been to many accidents before, but this would be my first fatality. Would my training be enough?

The wreckage was unmatched to anything I had ever encountered. Had I not been told it was the remnants of a motorcycle, a sports car, and a pickup truck, I would have suspected that a trucker dropped a load of scrap metal onto the highway. That all three had tried to occupy the same space at the same time, and failed, reminded me of the laws of physics that seemed so important to my life just months earlier at the university.

Quite a crowd had gathered and police officers struggled to keep the curious away from those that had come to serve. The air was thick with sirens, shouted commands, the roar of generators, and the sound of metal tools working on metal, but it was the soft moan and the plaintive plea from somewhere within the tangled mass of steel that spoke to our hearts the loudest. A strong odor of gasoline hung in the air as firefighters stood ready with charged hoses while colleagues worked to free trapped victims—a subtle reminder that such work was not without risk. But few noticed.

We were well trained. We saw what we were trained to see and did what we were trained to do. Still, it was hard to work around the two bodies that lay on the pavement nearby, their lifeless forms covered by yellow blankets. But the dead would have to wait for the living, or those with the chance for life—it was part of our training.

The enormity of the work at hand, the rush of adrenaline, and the discipline that training bestows, however, was not enough to block a lady's anguished screams from our awareness. Two police officers struggled to restrain a hysterical woman from approaching the accident scene. She had awoken with a start in the dead of night knowing that her twin brother needed her. It was a frantic need and it brought her to this place.

"I know it's him," she wailed, oblivious to the reassurances and logic offered by the officers. "Please let me go to him."

The damage was so extensive that it was impossible to identify the models of the vehicles involved, or even their color for that matter. There was just no reason to believe that her brother was among the victims, and even if he was, there was nothing she could do.

"His name is Tom," she cried, pleading for a sympathetic ear. "He has blonde hair and a wonderful smile. He wears a medical alert bracelet—he's deathly allergic to penicillin."

With waning patience, the officers struggled to comfort her, but she was not to be comforted. Only the threat of arrest and physical removal brought silence to her quest, silence interrupted only by the occasional and heart-wrenching sob that could not be ignored.

Extrication was tricky business. It was a scene more reminiscent of high-school shop class than one perfected in the service of others. Saws, pry bars, chisels, hydraulic jacks and brute force worked tirelessly to undo what the physics of momentum and energy took only seconds to create. As we worked, the sobbing from the midst of the onlookers haunted us, and I could not help but be touched by the humanity of what we were called there to do.

I reached for the yellow blanket that covered one of the bodies in the street and felt a hand grasp my shoulder. "Don't bother," said the police officer in charge. "We checked them out. They're both gone."

Perhaps it was the training, or maybe morbid curiosity, but I lifted up the corner of that blanket anyway and peered beneath it. Indeed, he was gone; at least I thought it was a he. Massive head injuries left no room for doubt. I had seen death before, but never as violent and horrific as what I looked upon that night. And yet, I moved on to the next body, albeit with some reluctance.

A severely fractured leg was obvious on lifting that second blanket. He was a young man and couldn't have been much older than myself. I knelt at his side to feel for a pulse, sliding a silver bracelet away from his wrist. But there was no pulse. The bracelet, however, intrigued me. It was silver and decorated with a red cross. Turning it over, even in the dim light, I could read the words *Allergy* and *Penicillin*. With a trembling hand, I placed my fingers on his neck. The skin was cool and dry and had a spongy texture to it, but there was something else—distant and almost imperceptible, but it was there. He had a pulse.

Three men lost their lives on that street corner that night, but Tom was not one of them. After many weeks in the hospital and even more in rehabilitation, he returned home. And I continued my journey, relieved that the training did indeed work but with a subtle awareness, or perhaps hope, that there was much more. It was a journey that looked different than what I had anticipated while at the university, but that's the miraculous thing about a journey—you never know what wonders lay just beyond the distant rise.

From our earliest moments of life, we are surrounded by teachers; teachers that mold our thoughts, feed our expectations, and sharpen our potential. More often than not, we are oblivious to them and to the influence that they had in who we have become. Every once in a great while, we recognize when that teacher comes into our lives and we know that their lessons will change us forever. It was that way with Betts Unger, but sometimes the teachers are challenging and their lessons difficult. Such was the case with David Trasket.

David Trasket—Chief Trasket as he preferred to be addressed— was a forty-year veteran of the fire service and the senior instructor at the fire academy. Fire departments from all across the state sent their new hires there for the basic training required of all full-time firefighters. I had always done well in school and found comfort in the chemistry laboratory or mastering new facts from a textbook late at night. But the time spent at the university, in paramedic school, or even the weekly drills at my hometown fire department couldn't prepare me for what I would encounter during those six weeks at the fire academy.

The classroom work came easy for me but it was obvious that most of my colleagues struggled with it. You could almost feel the fear in some; fear that their jobs might be at risk. It was common knowledge that if you were to fail at the academy it would happen in the classroom. One man in particular touched me deeply. He was just a few years older than me but already had a large family. Trebber had always wanted to be a firefighter but didn't have the high school diploma to qualify for the job. It took him three years of night classes and several tries at the examination, but he finally passed his GED and won a job on his small town's fire department. His eyes were filled with pride when he started at the academy, but when he learned that there would be tests to take, that pride quickly melted away to reveal an uncommon sadness, one that pleaded silently for help.

Trebber looked confused that night at dinner when I asked him if he would help me study. He was a quiet man and far too polite to ask the question that was obviously on his mind, so he reluctantly agreed. Each night we would sit up late in the deserted cafeteria and review the day's classes. Soon we were joined by another classmate and then another, each intent on helping me make sense of fire science, pumps, hydraulics, and building codes. By the second week, our study group had grown to include half the class and by the end of our six-week stay at the academy, not one examination was failed.

If I helped my colleagues in the classroom, the favor was returned on the training grounds. There my greatest challenges waited—and Chief Trasket waited with them. He was a cantankerous man who taught as he was some four decades earlier. He was suspicious of new ways and resented the precious training time that was lost in the classroom. We would not learn firefighting from books he would tell us; it could only be learned from him. We would never need to know anything that he did not tell us. There were only two ways of doing things: the wrong way and Chief Trasket's way. "God," he would tell us, "doesn't make mistakes."

Nothing represented greater change within the fire service—and greater distrust in Chief Trasket's eyes—than advanced life support. His entire career was spent without it and they had done just fine.

He believed that you only required two things to provide for the ill and injured: a stretcher and a fast vehicle. The sicker your patient, the faster you drove. Every moment spent caring for a patient at an emergency was a moment of delay from needed hospital care and a dangerous distraction from important things, like fighting fires.

Chief Trasket was certain that he wouldn't like me long before my arrival at the academy. It wasn't personal; he disliked all paramedics. Paramedics could not become firefighters any better than firefighters could become doctors—it was just the nature of things. Every paramedic in his class represented less attention that could be provided to those that he could make a difference with. It was a tragic waste and he could not help but resent it. As the only paramedic in my training class, I would require special attention.

It was unusually cold that early spring morning when the class gathered on the academy training grounds for the first time. A new aerial fire engine had been brought from the city and sat parked in the corner of the parking lot, its massive outriggers fully deployed and sunlight glistening from the polished chrome that accented its every surface. The giant ladder rose steeply from the bed of the truck and extended to its full one hundred-foot length.

In a booming voice, Chief Trasket told us that our first exercise would be to climb to the top of the ladder. Once there, we were to use a leg lock to secure ourselves to the ladder and extend our arms above our head for one minute. Just in case we did not pay attention in class on how to do a leg lock, we would wear safety belts and fasten ourselves to the top of the ladder. It was an optional exercise, he told us. Those deciding not to participate would use the time to pack for our return trip home. I was certain he was speaking directly to me.

When you think of firefighting, thoughts of ladders can never be far away. I had even come to terms with the realization that I would have to deal with ladders at the academy—I just hadn't thought it would be that soon or that the ladder would be so high. It wasn't that I was afraid of ladders; it was that I didn't know. My only experience with ladders had been the annual cleaning of the gutters at home—a chore that I admittedly dreaded. I didn't know what to expect. It was within that unknown that fear thrived.

I took some comfort in the fact that none of my colleagues seemed all that eager for the task at hand either. However, if any of them were afraid, I couldn't see it in their eyes. I wondered what they could see in mine. I felt confident though that watching others accomplish the assignment would help me face the unknown.

"Paramedic here," Chief Trasket said, "is going up first. It's a little windy today, so we'll see how he does before we risk any firefighters."

I stood, stunned by his words, certain that I had misunderstood them. I studied his face for the hint of a smile or the slightest suggestion that he was joking, but this was not a man that smiled, at least not in my experience with him. Every pair of eyes was fixed on me and for the first time I saw worry and concern in their gaze. In some, I even saw fear—not for themselves, but for me.

"Chief," one of my classmates spoke up. "Why don't you let one of us that have done this before go first? The new guys will learn more if they know what to expect."

"He doesn't have to go up," Chief Trasket defended. "He has a choice. He can either quit or start climbing. Either way, I think we are all going to learn something about paramedics today."

If it was my choice to make there would be little time for contemplation. A pair of hands set to work on the closures of my jacket while another tightened the strap under my chin that held my helmet in place. Yet another pair of hands reached around me to cinch tight a safety belt that had been placed around my waist.

"Don't look down," a hushed voice whispered into my ear. "Keep your eyes focused on your hands; take it one step at a time, and you'll be fine. You're not going to fall."

It was Treber's voice.

"Remember this," he went on, "if you get into trouble, just hook on with your belt and I'll come up and get you."

The absurdity of the situation was not lost on me as I climbed that ladder. We didn't have aerial trucks in my hometown fire department. We didn't need them. The tallest structure in town was barely three stories high. The most use our ladders ever saw was in putting up the holiday lights at Christmas time.

Treber's words played over and over again in my mind—they too seemed absurd. Of course, someone is going to look down when you tell them not to. Surprisingly, my glance down that ladder did not make me feel more anxious. Perhaps that wasn't possible. It was like looking back on a path just traveled—the rungs below a record of experiences passed while so much lay ahead. At the foot of the path stood my classmates—strangers actually—with their gaze fixed upward. While I didn't understand it at the time, they stood there for me. They wanted my journey to end in success, perhaps more than I wanted it for myself.

It was an unsteady journey. The appearance of stability that the huge apparatus offered on the ground melted away like a mirage the higher I climbed. With each step, the ladder would pitch forward and then backwards, its arc increasing in amplitude the closer I approached the top. Indeed, it was a windy day. I hadn't noticed it on the ground but its cold bite was hard to ignore as it subtly nudged the ladder from side to side.

It's amazing how much thinking can be accomplished in a hundred feet. Perhaps I had a made a mistake—learning skills that I would never use nor be likely to master. Perhaps the answers I sought could not be found in the fire service.

Approaching the top of the ladder, I found comfort in Treber's advice. With each step upward, I focused on my gloved hands—watching the fingers tighten around each aluminum rung, feeling the firmness within the grasp, and listening to the subtle sounds of leather against metal. Somewhere in that focus, the thinking stopped. I could feel the answers to questions that were no longer important. It is a strange place to feel peace—standing atop a hundred-foot ladder with arms raised above your head. Aware of distant clapping and cheering far below, everything seemed so clear that spring morning. Never again would I question the wisdom of the journey, but rather cherish the miracles that can be found along the way when we are ready to see them.

The weeks that followed were filled with many challenges—search and rescue, hazardous material, rappelling, and advanced firefighting techniques—and I always found myself at the head of the line. I always found Chief Trasket there as well. He was relentless in his pushing, prodding, and exploiting the weaknesses he found in others. There was much to exploit in me. Although I didn't look for it, I always found something else in those lines—the awareness that I was never alone and people determined that I would not fail.

There comes a time when we discover that what we know, what we have been taught, is not enough. We discover that there is something more, even though we probably do not understand what that more might be. It was an epiphany that came to me with a loud mechanical clanging. It was the alarm bell on the air tank that I wore on my back. I was almost out of air and had barely five minutes to make my way out of the burning building. Laying flat on my stomach, I wiped the front of my facemask with my glove, but it did nothing to improve my vision. The smoke was so thick that I couldn't even see my gloved hands. The crackling sound that once seemed to be off in the distance now was all around me and a deep orange glow appeared to float above me. The searing heat was overwhelming—much greater than I had ever imagined possible—penetrating the many layers of protective gear that I wore with shocking ease. Never before had I encountered such a difficult place. Never before had I felt such fear.

It was two days from graduation when the training class gathered at the old farmhouse some thirty miles from the academy. Occasionally, old buildings slated for demolition would be given to the fire academy for training purposes. It was a gift seldom refused as the opportunity to experience live fire in a training setting was both rare and invaluable. We would enter the house in teams of two—one trainee and one instructor. I never gave it a second thought that I would be the first to encounter the challenges that waited inside, but I was clearly taken aback when Chief Trasket approached dressed in full protective gear. He would be my teammate.

We entered that old house together with me in the lead holding the nozzle of the charged fire hose. Chief Trasket stood directly behind me, his hand clamped firmly on my shoulder. Already smoke was drifting down the staircase from the second floor, spreading out along the ceiling above us like waves across a pond. It was like climbing through a cloud as we ascended those stairs and by the time we made it to the top, only a small swath of visibility hung a foot above the floor. It was the space from which firefighters practiced their trade and through which we crawled in search of fire.

Every now and then Chief Trasket would stop to point something out about the alien world in which I found myself. His voice was muffled by his facemask and difficult to understand, but it seemed less gruff than I had grown accustomed to. I found his presence strangely comforting and the irony of that awareness was not lost on me. Even when the cloud of smoke completely enveloped us and I could not see him, I could feel his hand and hear his breathing. The air masks we wore betrayed not only our presence, but also our state of being. Every breath was loudly audible. His were slow and measured while mine were deep and rapid.

It is a powerful moment when you first realize you are in a room that is on fire. To be alone in that room is an awareness that touches a part of your existence that few come to know. The problems of yesterday and the worries of tomorrow—which seemed so important earlier—melt away when the present moment is encountered. Chief Trasket was gone. I didn't know how long he had been away from my side. I couldn't feel him. I couldn't hear his breathing. My outstretched hand couldn't touch him. I was low on air and was worried. The hose I clutched in my hand would lead me out of the building, but how, I wondered, would the chief ever find his way out?

In the instant my thoughts turned from myself to Chief Trasket, the fear that covered me like a blanket simply fell away. The bitterness I had tasted in my mouth for weeks strangely vanished. It seemed only seconds later that a hand once again grasped my shoulder and a muffled voice said, "It's time for us to leave."

We stumbled out through that old farmhouse door together. Despite the chill of the morning air, it still felt unbearably hot. After ripping the mask from my face, those first gasps of air were like deep breaths taken on a frigid winter's day. My gloved hands fumbled unsuccessfully at the buckle, securing the air tank to my back. Peeling off the gloves, I tried again, only to draw back in surprise when the hot metal burned my hand. A colleague sprayed us down with a waiting hose. The water hissed loudly when it struck our air tanks and steam rose from our coats.

As I struggled to catch my breath, Chief Trasket stomped up to me and focused glaring eyes onto mine while standing only inches away.

"Were you afraid in there?" he demanded.

"Yes," I said without a moment's hesitation.

A hint of a smile, almost imperceptible at first, slowly appeared on that weather-hardened face. It slowly grew until there could be no mistake—David Trasket was indeed smiling. It was something that I had never seen in him, nor even thought was possible.

"Good," he said. "Never forget it. You are going back to a dangerous place, not because of the number of fires you will see, but because of the fires you will not see. You can't become good at something you will seldom, if ever, experience. I'll wager that most of your supervisors have never encountered conditions that you have seen today. But one day it will happen—a fire that nobody ever thought possible; a fire you will not be prepared for.

"Look at your helmet," he said emphatically as he picked it from the ground at my feet. The once smooth edges of the black resin material was pitted and deformed, partially melted by the heat. "It was bad enough to die in there. Always remember what it felt like. The books you have read will not help you. The wisdom shared by your teachers will not be enough. The directives from officers will fall short.

"Trust what you feel. Listen carefully for the voice inside and trust what it says to you. Once you know it is there, when you need it the most you will hear it the best."

I graduated from the fire academy two days later and would never see David Trasket again, but I would never forget him. I could not forget him. Our struggle had been so personal and so intense that his memory was seared permanently into the deep recesses of my mind. He lingers there along with his lessons, waiting for the opportunity to teach. Along my journey, I would discover that his lessons were not about fighting fires, but about the secrets of life.

"There are only two ways to do your work," an angry voice said to us from across the conference room table, "my way and the wrong way. Doctors don't make mistakes!"

The words startled me to alertness. It could have been old Chief Trasket sitting at that conference table. Many years had passed since my days at the fire academy, but the vividness of the recollection quickened my pulse.

"I don't make mistakes like this," the white-coated man ranted on, slapping the tabletop with his outstretched hand for emphasis, "and I won't tolerate being made to look bad!"

It was the most emotion I had seen from Dr. Christopher White-head since he became our attending physician some three weeks earlier. A senior member of the faculty, he was clearly nearing the end of his career. It was equally obvious that he didn't want to be teaching because he was incredibly bad at it. It was not surprising to overhear him in conversation with his colleagues about his annual thirty-day sentence supervising a medicine ward team at the Teaching Hospital.

Internship was barely a month old when Dr. Whitehead became part of my medical education and that of two fellow interns. Our educational needs were so great, our experience so shallow, and our hunger to learn so keen that we would have learned from anyone. Perhaps that was the intent, and if it was, it was a hypothesis that would be severely challenged during those four weeks in August.

Even the terror that gripped our early days as doctors wasn't enough to thwart the incredible boredom that stalked us during morning rounds. No doubt, he taught as he had been taught, perpetuating the traditions of medical education from ages past. He was fascinated with statistics and the medical literature, the theoretical often taking precedence over the practical. It was a contradiction that frustrated young doctors. Our patients lived in the practical world and cared little about the theory of cure.

Morning rounds never changed much from day to day, filled with inescapable droning lectures that proved as powerful as the hypnotics that we prescribed for our sleepless patients. Emma Mae Ferris would change that.

Emma Mae was an eighty-four-year-old lady who lived alone in a small house not far from the Teaching Hospital. She was the definition of independence. She kept her home spotless and the garden that she tended was the pride of the neighborhood. Her family had long earlier surrendered the battle that she should not live alone. A favorite nephew stopped by every day to check on her, but he was out of town the day that Emma could not walk. The pain was just too great. Knee pain was not unusual for Emma, but it was something that she would not allow to keep her from her garden. That morning, however, she could not rise from her bed. When morning became afternoon and evening stretched into night, she reluctantly surrendered control of her world and called the ambulance from her bed.

In the emergency room of the Teaching Hospital, she would howl in pain whenever her knees were touched and then sink into a pool of embarrassment at having made such a fuss. She was always happiest when she could pass through life unnoticed and hated being the center of attention. With great difficulty and painstaking care—a difficult commodity in a busy hospital—x-rays were obtained of her knees. She had horrible osteoarthritis. No cartilage could be seen in either knee and bone rubbed against bone with every movement. Her doctors marveled at how she had been so active with such extensive disease.

While arthritis is seldom a problem that warrants hospitalization, her pain was so severe she was admitted to the medical service at the Teaching Hospital. While a colleague was responsible for her care, the entire team would see her every morning on rounds. She was a stoic lady and it was often difficult to assess her true level of pain. She didn't want her young doctors to think they weren't helping her. Our visits seemed more powerful than the narcotics and anti-inflammatory medications she was prescribed, her face beaming from the attention and the opportunity to learn something about each stranger that stopped by her room. Each day her pain lessoned and on the fifth hospital day, she felt more than ready to return to her home and her garden.

"What do you mean she can't walk?" her doctor said in disbelief to Emma Mae's nurse that sought us out while waiting for morning rounds to start.

"Just what I said, doctor," the nurse replied. "It took three of us to get her into a chair. That sweet old thing isn't walking anywhere!"

We rushed to Emma Mae's room and sure enough, found her sitting in a chair, her legs hanging limply like those of a Raggedy Anne doll. She had a broad smile on her face and seemed amused at the concerned looks on everyone's faces.

Her doctor examined her legs, lifting one and then the other, and shook his head in disbelief as each dangled lifelessly in his grasp. "Mrs. Ferris," he said softly, "why didn't you tell us you couldn't walk?"

"Why I did," she said with confusion in her voice. "That's why I came to the hospital."

"But you said it was because your knees hurt," the young doctor insisted.

"They did," Emma Mae agreed, "but they don't hurt anymore."

"Exactly," her doctor said with a loud sigh as if proving a point to a skeptical child.

"But I still can't walk, honey," she whispered as she placed her hands on her doctor's shoulders and peered into his eyes.

It was a slow walk back to the conference room and I pretended not to notice the tears welling up in my colleague's eyes. In those early days, we lived in fear of making a mistake. It was always with us and at times, the fear was almost overwhelming. We would lay awake at night and worry about the orders we had written the day before. What if we missed something?

"What do you mean, she can't walk?" the senior resident asked with wide eyes. "Does she have back pain?"

"Not a bit," the young intern insisted. "I just finished thumping on her back. Nothing!"

"So what's going on with her? Do you think she has had a stroke?" the resident asked, half-thinking out loud and half-asking.

"No," Emma Mae's doctor said thoughtfully, "a stroke wouldn't affect both sides. I'm worried that she has cord compression."

"Then you had better get a scan," his supervisor advised, "and get it ordered before Dr. Whitehead shows up."

It was good advice, but we all realized it was too late when our attending strode into the room to start rounds.

"What do you mean, she can't walk?" Dr. Whitehead asked incredulously. "You're sending her home today."

He listened to his intern's report with obvious impatience, gesturing with a moving hand to quicken the pace of the presentation. When the young physician finished describing Emma Mae's physical examination, his attending physician just sat there and stared at him. It was a full minute—moments that seemed to last forever—before he would speak.

"Do you mean to tell me that it took you five days to figure out that someone was paralyzed, and only then after a nurse figured it out first?" he asked with a sharp edge of sarcasm in his voice. "There is nothing like surrounding our patients with the sharpest and the brightest."

We were all stung by the criticism, but the wound penetrated Emma Mae's doctor particularly deep. He sat expressionless at the conference room table and it occurred to me that he looked no different than the shock victims I used to care for at the scenes of devastating emergencies. As bad as I felt for Emma Mae, I felt worse for my colleague. It could have very easily been me sitting in his chair surrounded by the awkward silence that hung heavy in the air.

"Dr. Whitehead, I don't think anyone did anything wrong here," the senior resident finally said. "The extent of Mrs. Ferris's problems was hidden by her inability to tolerate a complete physical examination. She was just in too much pain. She screamed the entire time the radiology techs were doing her x-rays. And with the amount of pain medication she has required, we were reluctant to try to get her out of bed before today.

"Maybe we could have detected the paralysis a day or so earlier, but that doesn't change the fact that she has it or the need to figure out what is wrong. We were just discussing that when you walked in this morning. Even though she has had no complaints of back pain, I agree with her doc's concern for cord compression and his plans on getting a thoracolumbar CT."

Dr. Whitehead adjusted his glasses and looked at the senior resident. "Are you defending her doctor or yourself?" he asked quietly. "If we are indeed talking about cord compression, then delay of diagnosis is not a minor issue. The longer the neurological deficit persists, the less reversible it will likely be."

It was early evening before I realized I hadn't seen Emma Mae's doctor since morning rounds. I hadn't known him long—certainly not long enough to call him friend—but internship tends to forge a closeness more akin to family, and I was concerned by his absence. After many minutes searching, I found him standing in a darkened solarium gazing out over the city that was bathed in the golden light of the setting sun. It was uncommonly beautiful and almost seemed wasted on a day that had gone so very badly.

"Are you alright?" I asked my colleague.

If he heard me, he didn't acknowledge my presence and I wondered whether I should be intruding upon an obviously private moment. He seemed to be off in a distant place but I knew he wasn't far away. I knew that he was with an elderly lady who couldn't walk.

"Are you alright?" I asked again.

"She has cancer," he said without moving his gaze from the sunset. "Tumor is compressing the cord at several thoracic vertebrae. There's no boney destruction, which probably explains why she didn't have back pain. But the CT also shows she has tumor everywhere. The radiologist thinks it looks like lymphoma.

"I just told her. She doesn't want anything done. She just wants to go home and sit on her porch and look at her garden. I told her that her garden couldn't cure her, but that maybe we could if she stayed in the hospital. She looked at me like I was a confused child that had a lot to learn. It was the second time today I was made to feel like a child."

"You didn't answer my question," I prodded. "Are you alright?"

Turning his face toward me, he offered a weak smile. "I'm fine," he said, "but thanks for asking. You're the only one that has. Actually, I've been standing here thinking about quitting."

"Why would you do that?" I asked, astonished. "You didn't do anything wrong. Nothing you did or didn't do changes Emma Mae's diagnosis. To give up four years of medical school after the first bump—of what I am sure will be a long and bumpy road for both of us—just doesn't make sense."

"I cried this morning," he said with more than a little reluctance.

"So," I said, "it's called being human. It's nothing to be ashamed about."

"Yes, I believe it is," he said with such sadness it would not have been difficult to find a tear in my own eyes. "Dr. Whitehead was so upset this morning. At first, I couldn't blame him, but even if I did screw up, he seemed more concerned about himself than Emma Mae. He's one of the giants in this hospital that we came to learn from and to be like. Sitting in rounds this morning, I realized I didn't want to become like him and it sort of hit me hard.

"But something hit me much harder. It was too late; I had already become like him. My tears this morning were not for my patient but for me. How can I go on knowing that about myself?"

In college, I encountered words from the knowledge of others.

In medical school, I heard words based on tradition and scholarship. In residency, I grew accustomed to words that came from experience, and far too often from the ego. These were words from the heart—something that seemed rare and precious in the world of medicine—and they touched me deeply. I stood with him for many minutes watching the final moments of the day melt into the night sky. There was nothing more to say so we stood in silence. In that silence, we learned much about each other and about ourselves.

A large part of rounds the following morning was spent with our medical team crowded into Emma Mae's room. Dr. Whitehead couldn't accept her decision to leave the hospital. He knew what was best for her even if she didn't and he tried to convince her of that. She wasn't buying any of it. In frustration, he turned to Emma Mae's nephew who had come to the hospital to take her home and appealed for his intervention.

"Sometimes," he suggested, "elderly people are not capable of making important life decisions and it is up to their families to protect them and do the right thing. I can't cure your aunt if she doesn't stay in the hospital."

"Doctor," the nephew replied with a smile, "I'm sure you mean well, but my aunt knows a great deal about life and seems to understand things that are beyond my ability to comprehend. But I don't have to understand. She knows what is best for her and I'm going to help her find it."

As we prepared to leave, Emma Mae reached out her hand toward her young doctor. Grasping it, he knelt beside her wheelchair and with a breaking voice said, "I'm sorry we couldn't help you."

"Oh, honey," she exclaimed, "you have helped me so much. You took away my pain. You have given me today."

She smiled at his bewildered look and placed her hand ever so gently on the side of his face, peering intently into his eyes. "Don't look so sad," she said, "be happy for me. You don't think I have much time, but you're wrong. I have a lifetime. None of us know what tomorrow will bring and that uncertainty can be a precious gift if we make use of it. That which is making you feel sad has reminded me that our stay here is brief and that we need to make the most of every day.

"While many have not discovered it, or maybe just don't see it when they are looking at it, we all have a special place where we feel at peace and have a sense of being part of something vast and wonderful. For me that place is my garden. The stillness there connects me with everything that has ever been and will ever be. But as special as that garden is to me, too much of my time there is distracted by what I need to do tomorrow, what happened yesterday, or that pain in my knee. But when we truly know and live our lives like there is no guarantee of tomorrow, we start to see the beauty and experience the power that can only be found today. Can you imagine how wonderful my garden is going to be every day of the rest of my life? You have given me time to appreciate today and I am very grateful."

I had been in many patient rooms while on rounds during medical school and my short tenure as a doctor, but I had never encountered anything like I had in Emma Mae's room that day. In that instant, I realized there was more, much more, to medicine than we had been taught or even considered possible. I had spent years learning everything I could about curing, but in the span of mere moments, I realized that curing wasn't enough; that there had to be more. And while I did not understand it, I knew that the more was healing.

Dr. Whitehead knew all about cure, but like most physicians, he knew little of healing. The startling realization that there was a profound difference between the two swept over me with the suddenness that a struck match can bring light to a dark room. Dr. Whitehead wasn't our teacher that day; neither was our senior resident. Class was conducted by Emma Mae Ferris. Her teaching credentials were not vested in advanced degrees but a life journey spent open to all possibilities and the willingness to share. It was an advanced class, perhaps one too difficult for physicians grounded in logic, tradition, and the science of medicine. For those not yet ready to learn, the lessons would linger in our thoughts and experiences until special teachers would help us learn the mysteries of healing. Those teachers would be everywhere—in every patient cared for, in the worried faces of families, and in the tears of colleagues—and they would wait patiently with us until we were ready to learn.

For the second time in as many days, I saw tears in the eyes of Emma Mae's doctor, but today they were not for him. His tears were for his patient who touched a special place in his heart, a place as special as the gardens that spoke so softly to Emma Mae. And whether or not he realized it, he would never be the same. A seed had been planted that day.

Teachers of the science of medicine and of cure had been obvious in my life for several years, but it was in those hushed moments in Emma Mae's room that I first started to realize the teachers of healing had been with me far longer. The awareness excited me, both for the lessons from the past that suddenly seemed less random and less confusing, and for the extraordinary lessons that I knew would surely come my way.

David Trasket taught that day. He was right about trusting what you feel and listening for that inner voice. I heard the voice so clearly in that room. Once you know it is there, when you need it the most you will hear it the best. So too taught a teacher that once stood among a crowd gathered at an accident scene looking for her brother. What we understand is far less important than that which we have never considered. Betts Unger was there that day as well. The trails upon which we walked in search of birds and beauty seemed to lead to the same special place that Emma Mae spoke of. It was a place I had forgotten about and one that seemed strangely important for a life of healing.

Emma Mae was looking for more—more than a teaching hospital filled with traditions and expectations could provide—and she knew where to find it. The search for more can begin only after the awareness that something is lacking. It seemed so obvious that morning in Emma Mae's room. I suddenly knew I would find more—more than that offered by medical texts, more than that practiced by my mentors, and more than I had ever thought possible—and my patients were going to help me find it.

CHAPTER 3

The Journey to Heal

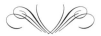

The most beautiful emotion we can experience is the mysterious. It is the power of all true art and science. He to whom this emotion is a stranger, who can no longer wonder and stand rapt in awe is as good as dead.

ALBERT EINSTEIN

For brief moments, our paths in this existence intersect with those of others. While our destinations may ultimately differ, for a while we travel together. It is in those steps shared with others that we can learn the most about our own journey. Far too often, we are oblivious to our fellow travelers or of what we might learn from them. The farther I walk on my path the more aware I become of the journey and find comfort, even exhilaration, in the understanding that the journey is more important than the destination.

The steps I have walked with medical students and residents have taken my journey through strange lands—wondrous lands filled with mystery, life-changing stories, and secrets of happiness—which few are blessed to see. The Buddhist proverb tells us that when the student is ready, the teacher will appear. Perhaps when the teacher is ready, the master will appear.

I never took a class on education during college. Teaching was never contemplated in medical school. Adult learning was not among the myriad theories encountered during the years spent in residency. So becoming a member of the faculty at the teaching hospital was both unnerving and bewildering. A senior medical resident one day, I awoke the next morning an attending physician. Knowing nothing about teaching seemed an almost irrelevant distraction to the machinery of medical education at the Teaching Hospital. How could I teach others to become a physician—a role that I was none too comfortable with myself?

My early days on the faculty were haunted by recollections of hapless, inept, and just plain horrible teachers that had crossed my path in training to become a doctor, although those earlier judgments suddenly seemed unfair and rather cruel. It was the exceptional teacher, however, that most captured my thoughts—those with the power to inspire and the drive to serve. My training years were filled with such giants and I longed to know how they had learned to teach. It was part of the path that I walked with my own students.

My teaching responsibilities would often take me to the VA hospital. It was a place I knew well, as much of my three-year residency in internal medicine was spent on the front lines there. It was a horrible place for curing.

There never seemed to be enough at the VA. The scarcity permeated every corner of every patient unit. Phlebotomists, transporters, and nursing aids—indispensable commodities at most hospitals— were rare sights at the VA. Medical students and residents would draw their patients' blood and push them in wheelchairs and gurneys to diagnostic studies. They would grow weary starting IVs, inserting catheters, and changing dressings—vital nursing tasks that might never have been accomplished otherwise. Morning rounds were conducted with blood pressure cuffs, thermometers, and by pushing an ancient set of scales as vital signs were rarely recorded on bedside charts. Evening rounds were conveniently timed to make certain that each patient had received a dinner tray. Scarcity was everywhere.

But there was also abundance at the VA—hidden behind countless unmarked doors scattered throughout endless corridors that few ever ventured down. Those doors would open every lunch hour and fill the cafeteria with a vast expanse of forlorn-looking souls, souls whose identification badges labeled as directors, administrators, managers, supervisors, coordinators, chiefs, and section heads. They were the neurons of the VA brain and from their consciousness would flow the institutional intelligence in the form of policies, guidelines, directives, and protocols—intelligence that seemed irrelevant to diagnosis and cure.

If the VA was a horrible place to find cure, it was a wonderful place to find healing, a distinction that might have slipped by unnoticed amidst the chaos of modern medicine save for the subtle lessons of special teachers that could be found there. The VA was a gathering place of diverse souls. The old farmer would encounter the student raised in the big city. The resident who graduated first in her class would spend time with the man from the hills who went to work as a boy and knew only how to feed his family. The ill man who was far from home found comfort in a faith that his young doctor didn't understand. It was through those differences that the journey was possible.

There would be a moment in each doctor's time at the VA when the eyes that looked up at them from a bed on morning rounds were not those of a patient but of a father, and not just any father, but their own father. A fleeting mannerism, a diagnosis, or perhaps the wink of an eye would trigger an almost mystical transformation from patient to someone who was so much more. Sometimes the moments were uncomfortably powerful. At times, young doctors would try to hide an embarrassing tear that clung stubbornly in the corner of an eye. Many times, you could feel the subtle longing for home. Those moments were inevitable at the VA and in their energy, however fleeting, could be found the capacity to heal.

That which made the pursuit of cure so difficult at the VA provided the greatest opportunity to discover healing. Nothing happened quickly at the VA. Tests and procedures did not happen on weekends or on the many federal holidays observed by the hospital. And even on weekdays, patient care would ground to a halt by three-thirty in the afternoon. It was the way that it had always been. Diagnostic studies performed as outpatients at most hospitals required admission at the VA and then often took days to complete. But the formidable obstacles that had become the culture of the VA spawned the willingness and determination of young doctors to overcome them. Through the countless delays in patient care came time—time to touch, to listen, to learn, to heal, and to be healed.

While my teaching assignment at the VA hospital seemed a burden in those early days of being an attending physician, there was no better place to learn about teaching. There I began to appreciate the journey and started to look for—if not expect—the unusual, the wondrous, and the impossible.

The memories of my first month as an attending at the VA hospital reside in a special place in my mind—amidst a collection of strikingly vivid images that chronicle those parts of our journey that seem to shape our lives the most. I can still feel the cool surface of the conference room table that I rested my hands upon that first day. Its surface was scarred from years of writing patient orders, history and physical examinations, and completing the myriad of forms that powered the VA system. Some of that writing I had done years earlier as a resident, but it was amazing to me how much I had never before noticed about that room. The large crack in the light fixture, the window that had been painted over, and even irritating squeak of the chairs with the slightest of movement; perhaps I had been too busy to notice before.

Abbey Bale sat with me at that table, along with the interns and students that would make up her ward team for the month. She had an air of confidence about her and just a touch of arrogance that one would expect of a senior resident destined for cardiology fellowship. But the discipline, focus, and logical thought that would serve her well as a cardiologist could be a liability in the chaotic world of the VA.

I looked at Sandy Fern with an uncomfortable sense of déjà vu. She seemed timid and fragile and looked like she could be brought to tears with the slightest provocation—unenviable traits for an intern at the VA hospital. Something seemed vaguely familiar about her. I felt as if I had passed this way before.

Months away from medical school graduation, the anxiety in Rajiv Cooker's eyes was obvious. A first-generation Indian-American, he was fearful of not landing the residency position that he and his family were counting on. His parents had sacrificed much in a strange new land in order to send him to the best of schools. He owed them success—a burden that seemed heavier than the demands of medical school.

It was Thomas Shipe, the junior medical student, however, that fascinated me the most. A few years earlier, he had been a construction worker. While I had encountered many disparate paths that had led to medical school, his was a first and I longed to learn more.

If I had thought that attending at the VA hospital would be just like attending at the Teaching Hospital, it didn't take long to discover otherwise. The lack of ancillary support services at the VA hospital added to the burden of its doctors-in-training. Being a good doctor wasn't enough. To make it through each day they had to be good nurses, technicians, and social workers. They had to be particularly good social workers. The nuts and bolts of patient care and addressing the insatiable social needs of our patients consumed so much of morning rounds that there was little time for teaching. Teaching did not happen at the conference room blackboard at the VA hospital, it happened through taking care of patients and sharing a part of their journey. Little did I know at the time just how powerful that teaching could be.

While many patients admitted to the VA were hospitalized through the extensive clinic system and some transferred from other hospitals, the vast majority of patients came through the emergency department. It is how Paul Zosterman would find his way to my ward team that early spring morning. He had been up all night in the emergency room—the wheels of healthcare delivery turned particularly slow in the emergency room—having been taken there by his son for concerns of confusion and agitation. He was rather cranky by the time he made it to a bed on the medicine floor, but not as cranky as the intern who was assigned to take care of him.

"Mr. Zosterman is an eighty-eight-year-old man with dementia," reported Sandy Fern on rounds that morning, "probably secondary to multiple strokes. He is billed as having altered mental status, but his examination doesn't appear any different than the last time he was seen in clinic. The only remarkable finding in the ER workup was a positive tailgate sign."

At one time, I would have found humor in her statement, but now, sitting at the head of the conference room table, it was difficult to suppress a frown. "Dr. Fern," I said in a soft voice, "for the benefit of our younger colleagues who might not know, would you tell us what a positive tailgate sign is?"

She sat silent for a few moments in a mixture of surprise and embarrassment before replying meekly, "It's when somebody drops a patient off at the emergency room and doesn't wait around to offer information or help. All you see of them is the tailgate of their car as they drive away."

"Look," she said with an edge of defensiveness in her voice, "this is a dump. Of course he's confused—he's demented. Next case! This man doesn't need to be in the hospital, but because his family doesn't care, he's going to wind up in a nursing home. I've been calling his son's phone number all night but no one answers."

"I admitted five patients last night," she said, her voice breaking slightly with emotion. "I don't have time to spend on people that don't need to be here. Do you know how long it's going to take to find a nursing home for this man? It's just not fair to the other patients, or to me."

I let Sandy vent for a few moments before venturing into the obvious conflict she was feeling. I felt her frustration. It hadn't been that long since I too was an overworked resident struggling with endless tasks that never seemed to make a difference.

"Sandy," I said with a sigh, "the short answer is there is nothing fair about the work we do. It is what it is. No matter what you do or how hard you work, Mr. Zosterman is still going to have dementia when he leaves the hospital. But that doesn't mean the work is unimportant or that you can't be of help to him. I'm not sure I can explain it, but your very presence is helping him, just as his very presence is helping you. You will learn something from every patient that you encounter, even those who you would rather not take care of. You may not recognize them, but the lessons will always be there. So my best advice is not to fight it, just let the day happen and seize each opportunity to be of help to somebody, even if you do not understand how it is that you may be able to help, and to learn."

Sandy remained silent and I wasn't sure she heard a word I said. Perhaps she found it best not to antagonize the attending—a survival skill learned in the earliest days of medical education—but more likely than not, her thoughts had already moved on to other pressing matters with other patients. But the plight of Paul Zosterman, and that of his doctor, would consume much of morning rounds for days to come.

Every morning we would stop by Mr. Zosterman's room and find that little had changed in the pleasantly confused man from the day before. His admission laboratory studies revealed a urinary tract infection and we had hoped that by treating it with antibiotics, his alertness would improve as it so often does in the elderly, but it was not to be. Every morning, Sandy seemed more frustrated. Days had passed and a social worker still hadn't taken on the task of pursuing nursing home placement. Phone calls to his son remained unanswered.

"It's just what I said it would be," fumed Sandy as we left Mr. Zosterman's room one morning. "We've accomplished nothing in four days. He's the same and a social worker has yet to see him. And it's just not the work. We need his bed. The ER is always full and there's no room for admissions.

"And don't get me started on that son of his," ranted Sandy. Clearly, nothing was going to prevent the young doctor from venting days of pent-up frustrations. "He hasn't even been by to see his father. What kind of person would do that?"

"But, Dr. Fern," interrupted her third-year medical student, "Mr. Zosterman's son is sitting just down the hall in the waiting area. I was going to tell you earlier but you didn't have time to talk before rounds."

Sandy Fern stood paralyzed by shock. "What did you say?" she finally managed to ask.

"His son is here," Thomas said. "I saw him in Mr. Zosterman's room last night. I've been seeing him all over the hospital the past few days. Every morning when I come to work and every night when I leave I see him sitting in the lobby."

"He's probably a volunteer, Thomas," Sandy insisted. They're everywhere in this place. What makes you think he's Mr. Zosterman's son?"

"Well," Thomas replied cautiously, "I asked him."

"You asked him?" Sandra asked incredulously.

"Sure," Thomas said. "Actually, he's a very nice man. I don't think he has left this place since his father was admitted. It sounds as if the nurses have known all along that he's been here and have been giving him regular updates. They even have his pager number in case he's needed. The strange part is that he doesn't spend much time in his father's room. It's almost as if he doesn't want his father to know he's here."

"Why would that be?" asked Sandra.

"I think you called it earlier. I think he feels guilty, but not for the reasons we thought." Thomas grew silent as his eyes lit briefly on each member of the team. Those eyes betrayed a story and an uncertainty as to how much to share. With a deep breath and rapt attention of his colleagues, Thomas continued.

"His mother died from cancer over a year ago. His mom and dad were married sixty-eight years and had never been apart. Even when it became clear that she would not survive the cancer, she wouldn't give up. His father's dementia was pretty advanced by that time and he needed almost constant attention. She wouldn't even take her pain medicine so that she could be alert to his needs.

"The day after he told his mother that she could let go, that he would take care of his dad, she died. He took a leave of absence from his work so that he could care for Mr. Zosterman. He does everything for him—cooks, feeds, bathes, and protects. The only time he leaves the house is to go shopping, and then he has to pay a neighbor lady to watch his dad.

"Now a year later, he has no income, his savings is gone, he's behind on his bills, and his job will not extend his leave any longer. He has no money for home health care and can't even afford to pay the neighbor lady anymore."

Thomas frowned and slowly shook his head. "As bad as all of that is," he said, "I think the worst part for him is the realization that he's not going to be able to keep the promise he made to his mother any longer. It finally hit him when his father became agitated and wouldn't sleep. He sat with him for two days and two nights and realized that he needed help, that he didn't know what to do for his father. I'm not sure that I have ever seen a sadder-looking man. He's been sitting here for days overwhelmed with guilt. I hope that there's something we can do to help him."

The awkward silence that followed was broken by Sandy Fern's unusually soft voice. "He's not the only one that feels guilty. I wanted so much to blame him for all of this that I never considered there was more to the story. I'm so angry that the nurses didn't tell us this, but then again, I never asked them if they had seen family. They probably thought we already knew about his son."

If there were lessons to be learned in that moment, they were silent and harried ones as the VA provided little time for contemplation and Bobby Perl was waiting just down the hall.

Bobby Perl was a sixty-one-year-old veteran whose long journey through the VA system was meticulously documented in the voluminous records that befit a government institution. Documents detailing previous admissions described him as uncooperative, noncompliant, and disruptive, labels no doubt penned by the hands of frustrated doctors and assuming the permanence of chiseled stone. It was a journey that Rajiv had read all about and even before meeting his new patient, he felt certain he would not like him.

Bobby Perl did not disappoint. Breathing made shallow by emphysema, and skin thickened and creased by years of weather and hard work, he was a cantankerous man seemingly intent on making everyone around him as miserable as he appeared. Hardly a month would pass when he was not in the hospital and he was typically discharged with the same complaints he was admitted with. Laboratory tests and diagnostic studies were routinely refused. He seldom filled the medications that were prescribed for him on discharge or kept follow-up appointments. When his breathing grew too labored, he would return to the emergency room, the severity of his lung disease always assuring admission to the hospital.

Rajiv, like the many doctors that preceded him, was convinced that Bobby had pulmonary fibrosis and he was determined to prove it. But his patient was determined as well.

"Mr. Perl," asked Rajiv as the team gathered around his bedside, "the nurse told me you wouldn't take your medicine this morning. Why not?"

"They don't work," his patient stated matter-of-factly. "Why would I take something that doesn't work?"

"But, sir, they're steroids. You need them for your breathing," Rajiv explained.

"They don't work," the determined man said as he shook his head from side to side.

"If you don't take them, how do you know that they don't work?" Rajiv asked, now with an edge of frustration in his voice.

"Did they give them to me the last time I was in the hospital, and the time before that?" Bobby snapped.

"Of course they did. That's how we treat emphysema," Rajiv said.

"That's how I know. If I was treated properly the last time I wouldn't be here now. I'm tired of you quacks coming in here making the same mistakes over and over again while your patients get sicker and sicker. There should be a law against this!" railed the angry patient between gasps of breath.

"Mr. Perl," Rajiv said with obvious concern in his voice, "you have to calm down. We just want to help you but we need your help to do so. We didn't stop by to upset you. I just wanted you to know that I was able to get a CT scan of your lungs scheduled today. It's going to help us figure things out."

"They were already up here to take me to x-ray," his patient replied. "I sent them away."

"Why would you do that?" Rajiv asked incredulously. "Do you

realize how difficult it is to get CT scans scheduled here? They were doing us a favor by working you in. It could be days before we can get another scan scheduled."

"I felt short of breath," Bobby said. "I'm not going anywhere until I feel good."

"Mr. Perl," the young physician-in-training said curtly, "you may never feel good again if you don't let people help you. Do you even remember the last time you felt good?"

"I was doing a lot better before you walked in here. I know that much," snorted the man who appeared much older than his sixty-one years. "You can help more right now by just leaving me alone."

I felt bad for Rajiv as we stood gathered outside Mr. Perl's room. His expression was much like that of a beaten puppy. "I knew he was going to be difficult," he said, "but I never expected anything like that."

"Mr. Perl has been raising hell in this place for as long as I can remember," observed Abbey, "but I've never seen anyone act like that before. One thing's certain: we can't help him by fighting with him. All that we will accomplish is to make ourselves angry and the day is hard enough without being hacked off all the time. No patient is worth that."

"I couldn't help but notice how frightened he looked," noted Thomas. "He reminded me of a small child who was scared to death of something that adults wouldn't understand. Maybe that's how we should approach Mr. Perl."

Sleep came hard that night. Paul Zosterman, Bobby Perl, and the dozen other patients on the ward team had preoccupied my thoughts the entire day and mercilessly followed me home that evening. The training years can be difficult, but my young colleagues were struggling more than seemed fair. But I didn't know how to help them.

Sometimes the answers that we search for cannot be found in our training and as I tossed and turned, I couldn't help but wonder whether *any* of our answers truly come from the years we spent in lecture halls or immersed in endless study.

The shrill ring of the telephone startled me, probably more than had I been asleep. While telephone calls in the middle of the night are seldom good things, during attending months they are particularly dreaded.

"I'm sorry to wake you, sir," Abbey said.

If only you knew, I thought to myself. "What can I do for you, Dr. Bale?"

"Mr. Gatwell is dead," she said. "We pronounced him at 3:05 this morning, about an hour ago."

If any remnants of sleep had been lurking in the recesses of my mind, they quickly vanished. Abbey's words jolted me to alertness with the efficiency of ice-cold water, but it was an unsettling awareness—I couldn't remember Mr. Gatwell.

Hoping for some clues that might remind me of Mr. Gatwell, I listened in vain to the awkward silence on the telephone many moments before surrendering. "I'm sorry, Abbey, you're going to have to help me. I can't recall Mr. Gatwell."

"I'm so sorry," Abbey stated, "you haven't met him yet. Well, I guess you're not going to either. He was just admitted tonight. I'm calling because you are listed as the attending physician."

Abbey's voice was different than I had grown accustomed to on morning rounds. It seemed less confident and there was a definite softness to it. I sensed that she needed to talk and since I didn't seem to have anything better to do in those early morning hours, I listened intently to her story.

Homer Gatwell was a name that many would recognize in our community. After the Second World War, the favorite son returned to his roots and invested his dreams and talents into a small farm. At eighty-seven years old, his fruits and vegetables were well known throughout the region and there was hardly a youth group that had not been graced by his generosity.

Few knew of his celebrity. Even his family was unaware. They were times seldom discussed and the mystery of those early years was gradually forgotten. There is not a detail so inane or trivial about a veteran, however, that it is not memorialized in the vast records of the VA. For those with the time and desire to explore, incredible journeys await discovery. Homer's would tell of service in the South Pacific, of torpedoes and a sinking ship, of heroism and saved lives, and of medals and honor.

It was a call from the chief resident that told Abbey to expect Homer. He had fallen at home earlier in the day and was taken to a community hospital where a fractured hip was discovered. He was to be transferred to the VA hospital for care.

Residents hated hospital transfers. Seldom did the description of the patient on the telephone match the severity of illness that suddenly appeared in a bed before them. Transfer patients typically bypassed the emergency room and the security it offered in detecting and managing unexpected problems. So it was with practiced apprehension that Abbey and her team waited for Mr. Gatwell.

Abbey was as relieved as she was surprised with the arrival of Homer Gatwell to the medical service of the VA hospital. He was the youngest-looking eighty-seven-year-old man she had ever seen. He could have passed for sixty-five. And he was the picture of health. Had his leg not been in traction, he would have looked out of place in a hospital. Despite an obviously painful injury, he appeared comfortable and denied any discomfort at all. He was a soft-spoken man with gentle ways and Abbey liked him immediately. It was his smile, however, that made him unlike any patient that she had ever cared for. She felt a closeness—one reserved for family and the closest of friends—that had never intruded upon her work before, and it bothered her.

She was also a bit perplexed for the urgency of Mr. Gatwell's transfer and felt bad he had been moved by ambulance in the dead of night. It could have waited until morning. He would certainly require surgery but it wasn't something that would happen quickly at the VA. She even had her doubts that the orthopedic surgeons would have time to see him before they started their busy day in the operating room. Misgivings aside, Abbey quickly completed the ritual of admitting a patient to the hospital, the history and physical examination being as reflexive as breathing to a senior medicine resident. She explained to Mr. Gatwell and his wife what they could expect in the days to come, answered all of their questions, and inquired about his desires in the event that his heart or breathing would stop during his admission. They were questions she had never grown comfortable with, but they were part of the ritual.

It was a rare night when the senior medical resident on call had time to sleep and Abbey knew it was too good to be true when she closed her call-room door behind her. Her head had barely hit the pillow when she was called to Mr. Gatwell's room. She found it just as she had left it an hour or so earlier—filled with family from the very young to the very old. Homer's face still smiled, but his eyes had lost their sparkle. His chest did not rise and fall and his lips were colored with a tinge of blue. Homer was dead.

The telephone line became silent. "What happened, Abbey?" I asked after a full minute had passed.

"I'm not sure," she said, her voice cracking with emotion. "I think he threw a fat embolus. All I could do was stand there and look at him because we had just made him a Do Not Resuscitate. I could have brought him back. I know I could have."

"How did the family take it?" I asked.

"Like they were expecting it," she said, sounding a bit bewildered. "His wife told me that he knew he was going to die and if he couldn't be at home then he wanted to be at the VA with his friends. And he wanted his family with him. That's why they all came in the middle of the night—because he asked them.

"Mrs. Gatwell told me they watched several of their friends' health fail and eventually die after hip fractures, and she tried to reassure him at the other hospital that it wasn't going to happen to him. He told her that he could see the light he had seen so many years earlier, but now he knew it was shining for him and it was time to join the others. She thought he was hallucinating from the pain medication, but he hadn't had any pain medication. This man snapped the neck of his femur in two and didn't have a bit a pain. Then he comes here and up and dies. I can't figure it out.

"Well anyway, thanks for listening," Abbey said after a deep sigh, "but I have to get back. I left Thomas with the family. I have to talk to them about an autopsy."

As I hung up the phone, it occurred to me that I didn't say anything about the ordeal that Abbey had just encountered. I offered no advice and shared no wisdom. All I had to give was time—time to listen—and I hoped it would be enough.

I arrived for rounds that morning laden with Danishes, bagels, orange juice, and coffee. The VA always provided food for the doctors-in-training after nights spent in the hospital on call, but many would question the definition that was used for food. Still, it wasn't the food that was always appreciated so keenly after a harried night, but that someone had thought enough to go to the trouble. Rewards seem few during the training years and a simple act of kindness often had a profound effect, if not being the subtle spark of awareness that theirs was a life with endless rewards.

While her team feasted on breakfast, I watched as Abbey slowly sipped coffee from a Styrofoam cup. She appeared to be off in another place. "Did you get any sleep, Dr. Bale?" I asked.

With an almost imperceptible shake of her head, she indicated that she had not, her gaze seemingly fixed on some marvel far off in the distance.

"Is there anything I can do to help, Abbey?" I asked in a whisper.

She again shook her head, but smiled and said, "No, I'm fine. I should be tired because I didn't sleep a minute, but I'm not. I met the most amazing people last night. Mr. Gatwell's family just left. I spent the last couple of hours with them in his room. I've been sitting here thinking that I spent more time with him dead than I did alive. The strangest thing happened. Thomas asked the family how Mr. Gatwell won his medal during the war. The whole bunch of them stood there dumfounded. He never talked with them about his service. They only knew he had lost friends. They never had the slightest idea he was recognized for heroism, but they weren't surprised. It's something that he would have kept private.

"Thomas offered to help them find out more about Mr. Gatwell's decoration, but they declined. It wouldn't serve a purpose. Nothing could add to their love and admiration for the man. He lived for the glory of the moment—an unblemished apple, a fresh cut field of hay, or sunset on the farm—and not those of the past.

"Something happened today that has never happened to me before. By every standard of medicine that I understand, I was a failure today. A patient of mine died and I couldn't prevent it. I couldn't even explain it. But all the family seemed to find was contentment. They were more concerned for me than for themselves."

Abbey paused for a deep breath, her eyes filled with emotion before continuing. "They actually thanked me. When they got up to leave, they all gathered around to give me a hug. The oldest son told me how much it meant to them to be able to be together when his father passed on. He told me how special it was to learn something new about a wonderful man who they had thought they knew everything about. He was their father, grandfather, and husband, and while nothing could increase their love for him, they were blessed with a better understanding of him and they would always be grateful."

We all sat in the quiet of our thoughts for a while before I offered an observation. "Perhaps Abbey, we need to find a new standard in medicine upon which to define success. Perhaps death isn't failure and there's something more important than cure."

Rounds seemed to go uncommonly smooth that morning. The number of new patients to see were few and their problems rather routine. It offered the team a much-needed pause, an opportunity to look beyond the urgency of signs and symptoms and to embrace what they found there.

With more than a little reluctance, I stopped the team outside of Bobby Perl's room. "I hate to end rounds on a down note," I said, "but Dr. Cooker, how is Mr. Perl today?"

"He's breathing better today after I turned up his oxygen to four liters," Rajiv said. "It is pulmonary fibrosis and it's worse than we suspected. The high resolution chest CT confirmed it."

"You got the CT?" I asked with a little disbelief. "He agreed to it?"

"Yes," Rajiv smiled, "and he even agreed to see the chest surgeons and is going to consent to an open lung biopsy. He might be a candidate for a lung transplant. It may be his only option at this point."

"I'm truly impressed, Rajiv," I said. "How do you ever manage to do this? He practically threw us out of his room yesterday."

"The credit doesn't really belong to me, sir," Rajiv said. "It was something that Thomas said yesterday on rounds. He commented on how frightened Mr. Perl looked. He was right. I've been in that room so many times but never actually took time to look at Mr. Perl. I was always too busy fighting with him. He looks terrified.

"I couldn't get that possibility out of my mind yesterday and started feeling downright guilty about the way I've been treating him. Can you imagine what it must be like not to be able to catch your breath, to spend every hour of the day like that? So I marched into him room yesterday and told him I knew he was frightened because I would be if it was happening to me. I told him that reality couldn't produce anything as horrible as that which we can imagine and that the CT scan couldn't reveal anything as frightening as what had been stealing peace from his life for too long.

"Mr. Perl and I talked about his two choices. He could go on as he has and deal with fear every day alone, or we could find out what was wrong and work with the problem together. No matter what happened, I promised Mr. Perl that we would help him through it. And it worked. He let me schedule the CT and I went down with him. I think last night was the best night he has had in the hospital for months. He even got along with the nurses. I've never seen such a change in a person."

"Do you really think he's changed, Rajif?" I asked without expecting an answer. Maybe he wasn't the one that was changed."

"I don't follow you," claimed Rajiv with a blank look on his face.

"Sure you do," I said. "Otherwise, you never would have been bothered by what Thomas observed and you wouldn't have returned to his room. Isn't it amazing that when you changed the way you looked at Mr. Perl, Mr. Perl seemed to change? I think you stumbled on a lesson that can help us all become better doctors. Thank you for that."

Rounds had been over for a couple of hours when I wandered through the conference room with a cup of coffee in my hand. Thomas was so focused on the patient write-up he was working on that he jumped a little when I sat down next to him at the conference table. "Sorry, Thomas," I said. "I didn't mean to startle you."

"You've had quite a day or two," I said, peering intently into his eyes. "I just wanted you to know how excellent your work has been. You've made a big difference to your team, something that I seldom see from medical students."

Clearly embarrassed, he looked away and said, "I haven't done anything. I wish I could. Dr. Fern is always so busy and looks so tired that I'd like to be more of a help to her, but I just don't know how."

"You haven't done anything?" I asked in surprise. "What about Mr. Zosterman and that magic we just saw with Mr. Perl? Do you think that would have happened had you not helped your colleagues see the person wearing the gown? And Mr. Gatwell—I just have to ask you—how in the world did you learn about his military service?"

A broad smile crept across Thomas's face and for a brief moment, he looked much too happy to be a medical student. As quickly as it appeared, however, the smile faded back into the darkness that we seldom notice but have grown accustomed to in teaching hospitals. He slowly shook his head and said, "After two years of medical school, you would think I would have figured out what information is important in patient care and what's not, but I obviously haven't. I'm not sure that I ever will.

"Dr. Bale picks up an old chart and within thirty seconds can recite a patient's entire medical history. Dr. Fern just takes a glance at a medication list and can tell you all about someone's medical problems. I know I'm supposed to be concentrating on those things when I look through our patients' medical records, but I want to know something about the person before I think about what's making our patient sick. I like stories—always have—and I've got to tell you, there are some great stories in these charts. It's a shame really; all of the wisdom and experience that slips through our grasp just because we do not know the story behind the patient and never think to ask."

When the student is ready, I thought to myself as I sat there with Thomas. I wondered if he recognized the power in his words. "I understand you worked in construction," I said to him. "What ever brought you to medicine?"

"That's right," he said. "I needed a job when I got out of college and thought I would work for this construction company for a few months until I found something else. I was with them almost ten years. It's hard to look for another job when you are working full time and I liked the people and the physical work."

"What did you study in school?" I asked.

"My minor was in English literature, but," he said with a trace of a smile, "my degree was in theology."

"That's one I haven't heard before," I said, "why theology?"

"Well, I was thinking about becoming a priest."

My fascination with Thomas grew with his every word. "Thomas," I said, "this is one of those times when it's okay to tell me to take a hike, but may I ask what happened?"

"Sure," he laughed. "I met a girl and wasn't sure that a religious life was what I really wanted. I always wanted to do something to help people, but didn't know what. The company I worked for was large and I met a lot of people. They all called me professor because I had been to college and whenever someone had a problem, they always came to me for advice. I discovered that people always felt better when I listened to their problems. It made me feel good too and I began to wonder what it would be like to have the tools to really help people. I wound up going back to school and the rest is history."

"You certainly took the difficult road to medical school, Thomas," I observed.

"Not really," he replied. "Sitting in class and studying was a lot easier than getting up every day and going to work. Being older had its advantages the first couple of years, but now that we are working in the hospital, I'm not so sure. I have a good ten years on everyone on our team but yet know the least of anyone. It bothers me at times. I wonder if I wasted all of those years."

"Thomas," I said softly, "the time you spent before medical school was not wasted. It was the path that led you here and that journey is unique for each and every one of us. You learned a lot on that journey, and while you wouldn't learn about the science of medicine and cure until you got here, those experiences helped you become a healer. Today we saw it in the eyes of a man that looked less frightened than they did yesterday, in the relief of a son whose father doesn't always remember him, and in a family blessed by the heroism of a life lived well. And we saw it in the faces of young doctors that, perhaps for the first time, encountered healing. They too have been enriched by your journey."

As Thomas and I talked, Sandy Fern rushed into the room and rifled through some papers stacked on the corner of the conference table, only to sigh deeply and quickly scurry away empty handed. It was her third trip in a half hour's time and her eyes looked red and swollen.

"They call her the crier," Thomas quietly mumbled as if thinking out loud. "I wish I could do more to help her. She struggles so."

"They call her what?" I demanded, feeling as if I had dosed off in the middle of an important conversation.

"The crier," Thomas reluctantly answered after an uncomfortable moment of silence. "The other residents call her the crier. But I…"

That was it. That was what I had felt on meeting Sandy the first day of rounds—the remembrance of an earlier time, a time when journeys collided. We were interns together at the VA hospital, Alison Chung and I. She was known as the crier as well. The slightest stressor—an unexpected admission, labs not drawn on time, or the difficult question on rounds—would cause her hands to shake and eyes fill with tears. But she had a kind face and a warm heart and seemed determined to confront her demons. It made for a long month during my first winter as a doctor.

Rounds were always busy then too. It was not unusual for each intern to admit four or five patients every night on call. While they were all sick, invariably one would be extraordinarily sick—illness that would demand much time from tired doctors who had little to give. Despite days filled with too many patients, too little sleep, and too many diagnoses left unknown, morning rounds was always the best part of the day. It was a time to learn, but also a time to serve. It was the rare patient at the VA hospital that was not appreciative of their young doctors' efforts and morning rounds was more akin to visiting sick friends than the practice of tradition. More often than not, and regardless the diagnosis, each room would house a smiling face and it was easy to look forward to visiting the next room—except for room 614.

Room 614 was typical of most of the rooms at the VA hospital and contained four beds. In the bed closest to the window was Zach Hanover, a Korean War veteran. He had an above-the-knee amputation of his left leg due to service-related injuries, and while it occurred many years earlier, he was visited daily by chronic stump pain. After he didn't answer his telephone for a couple of days, his family found him on the bathroom floor where he had fallen and was unable to get up. He was hypothermic and had pneumonia when he was brought to the hospital. He was a gruff but cooperative man, except with his doctor, Allison Chung.

It didn't take the observational skills of doctors-in-training to recognize that Mr. Hanover didn't like Allison. While her timid ways and indecisiveness drove her colleagues to distraction, it was hard to imagine any patient not liking Allison. She visited each of her patients multiple times throughout the day, often at the cost of not completing her work until late each night. It was not unusual to see Allison sitting at the bedside of a patient listening to their story. Her cheerful morning greetings had no affect on Mr. Hanover; in fact, he would disregard her presence on morning rounds and would only speak to the senior resident or attending. He would refuse her examinations, ignore her questions, and reject her advice. Every day as the team gathered around his bedside, he would ask for a new doctor, and every day the attending urged patience and cooperation. Every day Allison left his room in tears.

If we were bewildered by Mr. Hanover's actions, his family was mortified, frequently stopping the team in the hall to apologize for his behavior. The look in his eyes was unlike anything that they had ever seen before, certainly not that of the man who cherished family and friends and taught Sunday school for over forty years. It was a man they didn't know and he frightened them.

As tired as we felt the day following a night of call, the next day always seemed worse. Even a good night sleep could not erase the exhaustion cultivated from the previous thirty-six-hour day. It was on one such morning that we stood outside room 614. Alison was already tearing up and nobody wanted to confront Mr. Hanover that day. But it was part of our journey and the steps that we all shared that day would forever change us.

Mr. Hanover was crying when we entered room 614, not the gentle sobbing that occasionally intruded into this world of aging warriors, but howls of anguish so keen that they cut to the darkest depths of a private soul exposing secrets that perhaps were never meant to be shared.

"Tommy died last night," sobbed Mr. Hanover.

The bed next to the door was empty. It had been occupied by Thomas Peterson for many days, and while his death had been expected for some time, it was something that young doctors never got used to. He had been Alison's patient as well. Although his lung cancer was beyond medicine's ability to cure, Alison spent more time with him than any of her other patients. They talked about everything—careers, family, hobbies, and life's favorites. A retired English teacher with a love of literature, only blindness from macular degeneration could still his voracious appetite for books. Moby Dick had always been his favorite. The smell of fresh-cut hay, the sound of the whippoorwill, and the taste of butterscotch pudding that his mother always made lingered among the memories that brought him a special peace.

"Yes, we know Mr. Hanover," our attending said softly. "The two of you must have become very close these past few days. We are very sorry for your loss."

"He was so afraid of dying, just terrified," Zach said, "and there wasn't anything I could do to help him. He didn't want to die, but if it had to happen I don't think he wanted to be alone when it did."

"She knew," Zach said, pointing a trembling finger at Alison, "she was here."

"Dr. Chung was here?" the attending asked in surprise.

"She showed up close to midnight," Zach said with a hint of disbelief in his voice. "She had a bowl of butterscotch pudding. It was still warm. She had a book with her. She must have driven all over the city to find it. It was Moby Dick.

"Tommy was really too weak to eat, but it only took a taste. I've never seen anything like it. A spoonful of pudding did more for him than any of the medicine that he was given. Then she sat next to his bed and read to him until he passed. It must have been close to four hours. He had been so frightened and discovered that he didn't have to be."

"I'm so sorry, Dr. Chung," he said.

With only a moment's hesitation and a couple tears of her own, Alison grasped Zach's hand. "You have nothing to be sorry for, sir," she whispered.

"Yes I do," he said softly. "I never thought I would tell this story, but you should know. It happened when I was in Korea. It was a horrible place, but yet I found some incredible friends there. I was never good at making friends, but now as I look back at those years, I realize that they taught me how, and they taught me well. It's amazing how something extraordinarily good can come out of the darkest moments of our lives.

"Our unit was assigned to defend some hill. We waited three days for reinforcements that never came. During the day, we huddled in holes that we scraped and dug into the hillside and waited in fear of the setting sun. They would come for us in the dark. They would blow these hideous bugles just so we would know that they were on their way. We set off flares on the first attack and stared in horror at what we saw in the light. The hillside was swarming with the enemy—they were like locust. We were vastly outnumbered and they could have taken us in a matter of hours that first night, but they didn't. After an hour or so of fighting, they would just stop and fall back. Just when you dared to think that it might be over, you would hear the bugles again. They attacked three or four times every night. Winning didn't seem to matter to them. Their main objective seemed to be prolonging the battle, and the horror that came with it as long as possible.

"Each morning we would call out to the other positions in our unit, but fewer voices called back than in the day before. By dusk of the third day, my buddy and I were out of supplies. He was my best friend. We went through basic training together. The two of us spent three days in that hole and never spoke. We didn't need to. We knew each other so well that words would have just gotten in the way. We were both terrified. He was afraid of dying, but I was more afraid of living, of living another night on that hill. It wasn't long after we heard the bugles that a soft thud came from the bottom of our hole. It was dark and you couldn't see a thing, but I knew what it was. I don't remember the grenade going off. I don't even know how many days went by before I woke up at an aid station. I never saw my friend again."

"How horrible," Allison said quietly, now sitting on the edge of Zach's bed, "but you have nothing to be sorry for."

"Yes, I'm afraid I do," Zach said sadly. "Everyone tells me what a wonderful person I am, but it's all been an act. I've even fooled my family. I've taught Sunday-school children about love and kindness while living a secret life filled with hatred and intolerance. Please forgive me, Dr. Chung."

"I'm sorry, Mr. Hanover, but I don't understand," Allison said.

Zack looked into Allison's eyes for a full minute before taking a deep breath and responding with slow, measured words. "The enemy on that hill in Korea, those soldiers who taught me how to hate, and everyone that looks like them that I have felt hatred for all these years, they were Chinese."

"Zach," Allison said with a smile, "you don't need my forgiveness. You need to forgive yourself, and once you do, I believe you will see the special soul that all those people have seen in you; the special soul that I see." With that, the young Chinese-American physician leaned over and softly kissed her patient's forehead.

We stood watching in shocked silence—intruders upon the intimacy of life—awed by the mystery and power of two journeys that collided before us. Most of us didn't recognize it at the time, but we had watched healing that day and it would forever change us.

"That's not a bad thing, is it?" Thomas asked.

His voice startled me back to awareness. I was still in the conference room sitting with Thomas. "I'm sorry. What's not a bad thing,

Thomas?" I asked.

"A doctor showing emotion," he replied, "perhaps even crying in front of a patient or a colleague."

"No, it's not a bad thing," I contemplated out loud, "although most of us seem to pick up that message somewhere along the road. We spend years in training, but we are not that training. We spend much of our lives examining, diagnosing, and treating, but we are not that who diagnoses and treats. We assume these larger-than-life roles of physicians, but that's not who we are—we are much more. Sometimes that real us shines through the illusion that we project of ourselves—perhaps as tender smile, an empathic ear, or yes, even a tear—but I have to believe this is the part of us from which healing comes.

"Doctors may have mastered the technology of cure, but we haven't cornered the market on healing. We can learn so much from others. The wisdom that is acquired along life's journey is phenomenal, and it's ours for the taking. You have discovered the power of your patients' stories through listening and being open to what you might hear. A story is no more than a chronicle of their journey. If we listen, we can discover how to become healers."

Like most of the students and residents that I have had the privilege to work with over the years, I've lost track of Abbey, Sandy, Rajiv, and even Thomas, but the part of my journey that I shared with them has made me a better physician. They had encountered the wonders that could be found in their patients' lives and much like preparing an omelet, once the egg's shell has been cracked, there is no going back. There was much to find on the journey that we shared with those remarkable veterans—the students among us found teachers, the teachers found masters, and we all found healing.

CHAPTER 4

Spiritual Referral

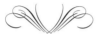

Footfalls echo in the memory down the passage which we did not take towards the door we never opened into the rose-garden.

T.S. ELIOT

When you examine the lives of the most influential people who have ever walked among us, you discover one thread that winds through them all. They have been aligned first with their spiritual nature and only then with their physical selves.

ALBERT EINSTEIN

The drumming of the pileated woodpecker reverberates through the hardwood forest and brings a smile to my face. I had never seen one before coming to this place. I hear so much in the quiet of these woods. It is here that my teachers speak to me most clearly, often in words spoken many years earlier, words that have lingered somewhere in my soul yearning for the understanding nurtured by the contemplation made possible in such a special place.

We are destined to encounter special souls on our journey—souls to guide us, teach us, and even protect us. On rare occasions, these guides introduce us to the singular teacher—masters of life that take us by the hand, and the heart, and lead us to extraordinary wonders and epiphanies of understanding. Herb Sefla was one such guide during my early days as a doctor.

Everyone knew Dr. Sefla at the Teaching Hospital. He was one of our giants. His name was prominent in the medical literature, stemming from an age when publishing journal articles was driven by the desire to share wisdom rather than achieve academic advancement. He was a pioneer in oncology, one of the first to use chemotherapy in the treatment of leukemia. I was both excited and apprehensive to discover him as one of my attending physicians early in my internship at the Teaching Hospital—excited by what this legend might teach but apprehensive about the powerful egos that I had already found in medical education, an ego that this senior professor must surely possess.

He was a big man who towered over most everyone in the room. His booming voice, firm handshake, and piercing eyes exuded confidence and discipline. There could be no doubt who was in charge when he was in the room. Of his many traits, however, I did not see ego and it surprised me.

Dr. Sefla trained in the very same teaching hospital that he now practiced in and taught, some five decades before I first walked through the doors. It was back in the days when physicians would start their practices after only one year of internship following medical school. Like most of his contemporaries, he hung up a shingle in the community in which he was raised and started a solo practice of medicine. For nine years, he sutured lacerations, delivered babies, and cared for the friends and neighbors of his parents and grandparents before giving it all up to return to the Teaching Hospital to become an oncologist.

Maybe it was those years that he spent as a general practitioner, but Herb Sefla practiced a style of medicine that I had never seen before in the specialist-dominated world of medical education. While formal with his patients, there was gentleness in his touch and softness to his voice. With every patient that he visited on morning rounds, he would always sit at their bedside a few moments before leaving. Words were seldom exchanged, but it was clear to me even in those early years that much was shared between patient and their doctor.

If his practice style seemed atypical for a faculty member of a teaching hospital, then teaching rounds were nothing less than astounding. One morning during rounds, he interrupted a discussion about the diagnosis of pneumonia to inquire about the necktie worn by a colleague of mine. He noticed that it wasn't tied correctly, an observation that was true more often than not when his inspection traveled from neck to neck around the room. It made quite a sight for those passing by the conference room door that day—a team of doctors in a busy teaching hospital practicing various necktie knots until they mastered perfection. It wasn't necessary for doctors to wear neckties Dr. Sefla noted, but if they did, then it was important to wear them well.

Every morning a member of the team would be invited to start their day at Dr. Sefla's tennis club. It was an invitation that no one was able to turn down and a game that no one was able win against an aging man more than twice our years. Lunch would always find one of us dining with Dr. Sefla. No matter how busy we perceived our day to be, we found that there was always time to eat and to eat well. As each day drew to a close, Dr. Sefla would invariably be seen with an arm around the shoulder of one of his young colleagues walking them to the faculty lounge. There over coffee would be discussed things of importance—family, friends, and hobbies—that had somehow become forgotten.

Herb Sefla taught more than medicine. He taught about life—not just the lives of patients, but also the lives that took care of those patients. His awareness that you could not be a good doctor if you were not a good person seemed a startling revelation in a teaching hospital. We would learn that taking care of ourselves and exploring the potential stored deep within our souls would enable us to provide more to our patients than we had imagined possible.

Barely a week had passed on Dr. Sefla's team when I became aware of a powerful sense of calm amid the haste and turmoil that defined life in the Teaching Hospital—almost as if my soul took a deep sigh of relief. As a senior medical student, I had interviewed at many residency programs looking for the ideal place to start my career. I was never truly certain just what it was that I was looking for, but by the end of my visit with most programs, I knew what I wasn't looking for. I had found programs that excelled in academic-centered medicine, technology-centered medicine, and far too many that had perfected ego-centered medicine. Somewhere between morning rounds and afternoon chats with Dr. Sefla, I realized what I had been looking for—and indeed had found—was patient-centered medicine.

If it was possible for a single discipline to rise above the many that possessed our thoughts and consumed our time in medical school, mine was oncology. I found the pathology of cancer fascinating and the impact that it can have on life to be unlike any other encountered in medicine. The days spent with Dr. Sefla rekindled that early interest. It had been a long time since I had felt so inspired. His was a caring oncology, one where technology and academia were tempered with love and touch was therapeutic.

I was not far into my second year of residency when I knocked on Dr. Sefla's door late one afternoon. It was a door that was always open and while every flat surface was stacked high with books and papers, his office always felt warm and inviting. He had become my mentor and I found myself drawn to him when contemplating a problem or finding fulfillment through a difficult diagnosis or a patient's smile. He couldn't have been happier when I told him I had decided to pursue a career in oncology. When I accepted an oncology fellowship at the Teaching Hospital—a position no doubt he had helped to arrange—the smile on his face reminded me of a proud parent. While fellowship was still eighteen months away, I didn't have to wait long before becoming consumed with cancer. At the Teaching Hospital, it was everywhere.

It wouldn't be long before my decision to dedicate my professional life to the care of cancer patients would be profoundly challenged. I didn't know it then, but the obnoxious shrill tone from my pager that disturbed medical grand rounds one afternoon would herald a haunting that would follow me through the rest of my residency. Carrying pagers while attending grand rounds was frowned upon by the Department of Medicine, but working in the Intensive Care Unit that month left no alternative other than not attending the mandatory conference. With every pair of eyes focused on me, I shrank from that conference room to find even greater discomfort waiting in the ICU.

It was Billy Grasper, who at thirty-one years old was my age. Nothing draws a resident's attention from the theoretical to the absolute more than caring for a patient their own age—even more so when that patient was ill enough to require hospitalization in the intensive care unit. However, when that illness was cancer, one was visited, if only briefly, by the specter of mortality. It was always an unpleasant haunting.

As cancer goes, few were more horrendous than the malignant melanoma that plagued Billy's life. Diagnosed some four years earlier, Billy was hardly concerned when told that the black spot that had been removed from his back was cancer. He was too focused on starting a family and demonstrating his worth to the law firm that had just hired him to give skin cancer a second thought. It was a problem that old people had, and even then, not much of a problem to get worked up about. He wasn't even that worried when a year later, a lump under his arm contained the same type of cancer cells. But when the scans showed tumors invading his lungs, liver, and even his brain, he began to question the career that seemed to consume his quest for happiness.

The specialists all exuded optimism and it was easy to share their enthusiasm and eagerly embrace their counsel. After all, he was young and healthy and the perfect candidate for cure. But cure was elusive. As one treatment would fail, there was always another doctor with new options and even greater hope. But the operations, radiation treatments, and cycle upon cycle of chemotherapy—each leaving his body a little more ravaged than the one that came before—did little to quell the relentless advance of his cancer.

The oncologist at the Teaching Hospital assured Billy and his family that all was not lost. Yes, he had an aggressive cancer that killed virtually everyone that encountered it, but this was, after all, the Teaching Hospital and they had something new to offer. The problem with chemotherapy, the doctor explained, was that the dosage needed to kill Billy's cancer cells would also kill the healthy cells, likely killing Billy as well.

After years of disappointment and dashed hopes, Billy's family was told that his answer and only hope for cure was a bone marrow transplant. Billy would receive a massive dose of chemotherapy, more than enough to kill the melanoma that had spread throughout his body. Unfortunately, the chemotherapy would make Billy ill and would wipe out his bone marrow along with his body's ability to produce blood and infection-fighting cells. But before Billy received the chemotherapy, bone marrow would be extracted through needles placed into his pelvis and frozen. Once the chemotherapy was finished, the stored cells would be infused back into Billy's veins where they would make their way to his bone marrow to replenish it with life.

Billy was the Teaching Hospital's first bone marrow transplant and excitement hung in the air like a morning's fog, and like a fog, it floated down every corridor and wrapped around every corner of the institution. The nurses that cared for him, the technicians that tended the monitors, and even the lady that cleaned his room knew that something special was happening in that corner room of the ICU. The doctors felt immense pride to be part of something groundbreaking. The oncologists were downright giddy with delight, so much so that one wondered if they knew just how sick Billy had become.

Billy was indeed sick, probably the sickest patient that I had ever cared for in my short career. It had been a week since he had received his chemotherapy and his transplant had followed a few days later. The toxicity of the chemicals that were administered to him was sobering and it was difficult at times to accept that it had been done in the quest for cure. Not a body system was spared insult. His kidneys had not worked for several days and his liver was failing. He was profoundly anemic and required transfusions almost continuously, transfusions that did little to stem the worried looks that came with every laboratory report. When awake, Billy would mumble incoherently and we found comfort in the belief that he was unaware of what was happening to him.

His nurse met me at the door of the ICU; the worried look on her face seemed to grow more intense with each passing hour. "Sorry to get you out of Grand Rounds," she said, "but look at these blood gases."

We had hoped that the sensor strapped to his finger measuring blood oxygenation was inaccurate, but the blood drawn directly from an artery in his wrist confirmed my worst fears. Billy was in respiratory failure and would need to be placed on a ventilator or he would not survive. It was a decision too important to be made on my own and within minutes, the supervising fellow and ICU attending had crowded into Billy's room with the rest of the team. Everyone was in agreement as the crash cart and ventilator were rolled into the room, although it was an uneasy agreement.

"Does anyone know his code status?" one of the residents asked. "Does he even want this?"

The question startled us, not because it was inappropriate to ask, but because none of us knew the answer or even had contemplated its need. Surely, his doctors would have addressed such an important issue with Billy before his transplant, but no such documentation could be found in a frantic search through his voluminous chart. His family, at his bedside almost constantly, had stepped away for lunch and could not be located for guidance. Without instructions to the contrary, we took Billy into the darkness of modern medicine.

I was quite adept at intubation, no doubt from the years of practice as a paramedic in the most challenging of circumstances, but I struggled to place the tube that would attach Billy to the ventilator into his trachea. Blood in the back of his throat made it difficult to see his airway, but with the help of the respiratory therapist and frantic suctioning, we were able to take control of his breathing. But it was a shallow victory.

Even with the help of the ventilator, it was difficult to improve the amount of oxygen reaching Billy's bloodstream. The monitor above his bed tracked a worrisome decline in his blood pressure necessitating even more medications to be added to the plethora of IVs that hung from the ceiling. Blood trickled from Billy's nose and oozed from every site where a needle had punctured his skin. Billy was dying and there was nothing we could do about it.

"No, he's not dying," said a firm voice rising above the tension in the room. It seemed to be more of a command than an observation. It was Billy's oncologist.

"Thank heavens his family wasn't here," he said.

"Now why is that a good thing?" I asked somewhat incredulously, the sleeves of my white lab coat soaked with blood.

"They might have told you not to tube him," the senior physician said matter-of-factly.

"I beg your pardon?" the ICU fellow asked.

"Look," the oncologist said with an edge of impatience in his voice, "this is what they signed up for. We need to see this through. The transplant was a huge success. Now we just need to support the patient until our treatment has had time to work."

It was an easier desire to express than to achieve. Every result rushed back from the laboratory looked worse than the one before. Three medications now ran into Billy's veins to keep his blood pressure barely above death. Even with the ventilator, his lungs couldn't provide enough oxygen to the rest of his body. His heart, once racing rapidly, now grew slow and irregular.

A radiologist technician rushed the stat chest films into the room and we crowded around the light box, desperate for good news. But we wouldn't find any in those x-rays. His lungs were completely obliterated by dense white shadows; perhaps pneumonia, but most likely, Billy was bleeding into his chest. We had no way to treat it.

The oncologist anxiously looked at the cardiac monitor. "Let's put in a pacemaker," he said.

The room, a beehive of activity, grew strangely and instantly quiet. Every pair of eyes set upon the oncologist, some in disbelief, some in shock, most filled with tears. The resistance was palpable and it mystified the cancer doctor.

"I don't understand," he said, looking about the room. "Am I the only one who wants to save this man? He's expecting us to cure him and we've done that. Don't give up the race just before we cross the finish line. We have to do whatever it takes to keep our promise to him. Nothing is out of the question—absolutely nothing!"

We had been in Billy's room working franticly for almost three hours and until that moment, I hadn't given what we were doing a second thought. Most of my days were like that—from the tedium of the routine to the exhilaration of the extraordinary—we had grown accustomed to acting without thinking about it. Seldom, however, was there much need for such thought at the Teaching Hospital—the needs of our patients always seemed to complement those of their doctors. Doing the right thing seemed instinctive, except perhaps at that moment. I never had to consider asking *why* before and that realization bothered me.

The painful silence that shrouded the room and the indecision that haunted my once disciplined thoughts were brought to a merciful end with the unusually commanding voice of my attending physician. Typically a soft-spoken man, he always seemed out of place to me in the ego-driven world of the ICU. He was an older doctor, his clinical wisdom no doubt forged before technology intruded upon the intimacy possible between patients and their physicians and the wonders that could be found there. He used words sparingly, as if conserving a precious resource, teaching instead by doing.

"No," he said, "Mr. Grasper has had enough."

The oncologist looked both bewildered and shocked. "I'm Billy's doctor," he insisted emphatically, "and with all due respect, sir, I'll decide when he has had enough. As long as his heart is beating, he has hope and we must try. Nothing that we do can hurt him, only help."

"We can hurt him a great deal," the ICU attending said softly, "and I fear we already have. Just because we can do something doesn't mean that we should. Death is not failure, not his or ours. You have given Billy his chance to get better. We can do no more, and in this unit, we will do no more."

Billy's oncologist stood in wide-eyed astonishment for a long moment, perhaps weighing the wisdom of challenging a colleague in such a public place. He turned to leave but paused briefly when his gaze fell upon me. If I expected to see contrition in those eyes, I found none, but there was a hint of disappointment and I wondered if it might be for me. He was a major figure in the fellowship program and soon he would become both my boss and my teacher. I too felt disappointment.

We did our best to keep Billy comfortable but no longer intervened when his blood pressure fell further and less and less oxygen found its way into his tissues. We watched as his heart rate slowed and its rhythm grew increasingly chaotic, and we watched—with his mother at his side holding his hand—as Billy completed his journey. If there was grief in his mother's eyes, there was also relief and something more. She spoke of seeing peace in her son's face, peace that had eluded him for many months and peace that she had feared he would never see again. And while Billy's doctors may not have understood, she was very grateful for that moment of peace. It was what they had been looking for.

Billy's death bothered me like no other. He haunted me. His visits often came at the most inopportune time—when meeting a patient for the first time, a moment of quiet after a harried night of call, when offering comfort and reassurance to family members, or when contemplating my future as an oncologist.

Everyone had cancer at the Teaching Hospital, or so it seemed, once I had chosen oncology as a specialty. Many of our patients did well, but there was much sadness. The young patients troubled me the most, the ones with children at home and lives not that different from my own. Mortality would never again be an abstraction after meeting them and the brevity of life became a daily awareness.

Many of my cancer patients would die during my last year of residency, but death was not a stranger to me—I had encountered it often along my journey. Despite a diagnosis that exposed the impermanence of life so vividly, their oblivion to the possibility of their own death astonished me. They were among the most ill prepared to face death than any of the other patients I encountered at the Teaching Hospital. New chemotherapies, innovative radiation techniques, and cutting-edge surgical procedures seemed certain in their ability to defy death, or at least the reality of it. Often it appeared that those with the gravest prognosis held the greatest expectations of cure, and the life squandered in treatment rooms and hospital wards saddened me.

If I was surprised by my cancer patients' denial of their mortality, that shown by their oncologists left me astonished. Death spares few in medicine—even touching the dermatologist and plastic surgeon at times—but it visits the oncologist with uncommon frequency. I always thought that oncologists would be better at dealing with death than other physicians, an assumption that was profoundly challenged in those days at the Teaching Hospital. Far too often I would find myself wondering whether the aggressiveness in which they attacked tumors had more to do with themselves than with their patients.

It was late in my third year of residency and the light that shone from the end of the tunnel was of such intensity that one would wonder if it was not a locomotive heading in my direction. The late afternoon sun streaming through the windows bathed the nursing station in a warm glow and somehow made the stack of paperwork that I struggled with less of a burden. It was spring and my thoughts would drift to earlier times that had made it my favorite time of year. The illusion of peace did not last long—consumed within the anger of the words that I became aware of across the table from me.

I had seen Jason Crosswell infectiously happy, fatigued to the point of exhaustion, awed by the unknown, moved to tears, and humbled by the opportunity to serve, but I had never seen him angry before and it startled me. He had been one of my senior residents in the early days of my internship and I owed a lot of what I had become to him. I marveled at his compassion and skill at relating to patients in their most difficult hours. His mastery of medical literature was second to none, but it was his understanding of people that made him a unique physician. I hadn't seen much of Jason since he joined the oncology fellowship at the Teaching Hospital and I was excited at the prospect of working with him again the following year.

"You still don't get it, do you?" Jason challenged the intern sitting next to him. "Your role on this service is to do whatever you are told and to do it without question. We'll do the thinking for you. In exchange, you'll leave at the end of the month a lot smarter than when you started."

"But I didn't do anything wrong," the young physician insisted as she fought back tears.

"Didn't do anything wrong!" Jason fairly shouted. "You asked Dr. Osgood's patient if he wanted the hospital chaplain to stop by for a talk."

"Yes, and what's wrong with that?" she demanded.

"Dr. Osgood doesn't do religion. It destroys patients' faith," Jason said.

"I'm sorry?" the intern asked incredulously.

"Cancer patients have to trust their oncologists implicitly. They need to understand that they might be too ill to make their own decisions and that we know what is best for them. If they think they are going to die, they may not agree to treatment. Look, you might have meant well, but you undermined Dr. Osgood in that room. If a minister walks in that room, Mr. Peterman might think he's going to die."

"He is going to die," she said bluntly, now with a touch of anger creeping into her own voice. "Mr. Peterman has metastatic pancreatic cancer. You gave the lecture last week. You know the nine-month survival statistics."

"Statistics are for us, not for our patients," the oncology fellow countered. "And Mr. Peterman has lived ten months after diagnosis. Dr. Osgood gave him that extra month. It's a huge victory."

"But at what cost?" she asked. "He's on a morphine drip that's barely covering his pain, he spends more time in the hospital than he does at home, he can't eat, and he can't even feel his wife's touch through the gloves she has to wear when he's in isolation. That man needs to be in hospice."

"Never," Jason exclaimed with a horrified look on his face. "That would be admitting defeat. There is always something that can be done. We do not do hospice on this service—never!"

The heated exchange turned many heads in the nursing station and a wave of embarrassment seemed to crash over the young intern when she realized she had been the center of attention. She hurriedly gathered her things before slipping away but the profound sadness that could be seen in her eyes could not be denied. I couldn't help but wonder if the sadness was for herself or for her older colleague.

I sat stunned. My paperwork forgotten, I could manage nothing more than to sit in silence and watch my old friend. Perhaps sensing my gaze, he looked up at me uncomfortably and snapped, "What?"

"Jason," I said in a hushed voice.

"What?" he demanded again. He was still angry but now seemed to be aware of it and that awareness appeared to embarrass him.

"Jason," I said again quietly while slightly shaking my head. It was all I could manage to say, although the question that burned in my heart must have been obvious on my face.

Jason stood to leave but turned and looked deep into my eyes. "We'll see how much you've changed this time next year," he said matter-of-factly before walking away.

Few words have ever troubled me greater or better described the silent struggle that had raged within me for many months. Sitting on a worn park bench that evening, the words replayed in my thoughts over and over again. While just a few blocks from my home, it was the first time I had ventured to the park since moving to the city. Life was always too busy and something seemingly more important invariably demanded what precious free time residency allowed. But that night something drew me to the park. Maybe the call had always been there, but for whatever reason, that night I followed it.

It wasn't a large place, but the heavily wooded floodplain of an adjacent stream gave the retreat an expansive impression. There wasn't another soul in sight and I sat alone in the quiet. It was so unlike the frenzy I had grown accustomed to, but yet there was something familiar about this quiet, like returning home after many years away and finding a childhood friend waiting. There was much to hear in the quiet—the rustle of leaves from a scampering squirrel, the faint whistle from the breeze passing through the branches of tress, the chatter of the chipmunk—and the more I listened, the more I could hear.

I heard the birds the best. It had been many years since I had last visited the marsh, or any place in search of birds, and there was a child-like thrill in finding them here. Perhaps they were the friends that had waited for me. I couldn't see them in the fading light of evening, but I knew they were there. Their songs filled the small woodlot that surrounded the bench upon which I sat and filled a part of me that had been feeling so very empty of late with an almost forgotten warmth. The flute-like notes of the wood thrush, the buzz of the nighthawk, the chatter of the wren, and the incessant call of the titmouse—they were all there, friends and teachers from my youth. It was something that Betts Unger had taught me—the ability to identify birds only by sound—and I was always amazed at how much you could hear in the quiet. I rediscovered quiet that night—chastened that it had always been so close and grateful for the answers that could be found there.

I had been waiting in Herb Sefla's office for better than an hour the following morning before he strode in with a coffee cup in one hand

and the newspaper in the other. Even before he had made it to his desk chair, he was in full conversation mode. He excitedly described the backspin that his tennis opponent had placed on the ball that morning. He marveled at the cranberry muffins the corner deli always served in the morning and how the parking garage attendant never failed to greet him with a smile. When his eyes fell upon mine, he grew instantly silent and the smile that always defined his face vanished.

"Bill," he said, "What's wrong?"

It was difficult to look him in the eye, but I was determined that that was how this conversation would take place, even if he noticed the tear or two I was trying my best to hide in my own eyes. I thought that I owed him that much, but in actuality I owed him much more.

"Dr. Sefla," I started, "there is nobody I respect more than you and the thought of disappointing you or making things difficult for you makes me sick, but I just can't do this. I know it's late, but I-"

"It's okay," he interrupted. "You don't have to say another word. I understand."

With those few words, I was released from my commitment to join the oncology fellowship at the Teaching Hospital. If there was relief, it was only momentary and quite shallow, barely lasting long enough for me to find a quiet place where I could be alone with my thoughts. For the first time since starting medical school, the future seemed uncomfortably uncertain. Residency would end in less than three months and I had not a clue as to what I would do then. Practice seemed most likely, but time was short and I didn't have the slightest idea where to look or who to talk to. I had spent so much time in training that it never occurred to me that one day I would put what I had learned to use, much less on how to go about doing it. I wasn't all that sure I would even be any good at it. Feelings of betrayal and guilt never strayed far from me that day and I worried about those that my decision would inconvenience. I feared that I had disappointed a man that had become more than a mentor to me, and that was the worst of all.

By day's end, I had been summoned to the department chairman's office. The retribution that I had expected all day—and was rather surprised that it had not yet come—was no doubt close at hand. The angry face I had steeled myself for in the forty-five minutes of waiting in a straight-backed chair outside his office door was strangely absent when I was finally ushered in to meet him. Indeed, he had heard about my conversation with Dr. Sefla that morning, but he did not appear angry. He did not rant, rave, or pressure me to reconsider. He did, however, ask me to join the faculty and become part of their practice when I finished my residency. It was an offer that would take me back to the park that night and a decision that would be found in listening to the quiet of the wood thrush, the breeze through the trees, and, of course, the titmouse.

In the blink of an eye, I was deeply immersed in the practice of medicine. While I had thought I was busy as a resident, nothing could have prepared me for the demands that private practice would ask of me. Life changed so quickly and so thoroughly that I didn't have much of an opportunity to dwell on the possibility that I wasn't good enough to be a member of the faculty. The point had become moot—good enough or not, I was a member of the faculty.

My office schedule filled quickly, not with patients seeking me, but with the myriad of souls that a medical school faculty practice attracts but who could not be accommodated by the established physicians in the group. In the early days, I often felt guilty that patients had come seeking the best and instead received me. To my surprise, most of those patients returned for a second and third visit and somewhere along the line, I became their physician. It was an even greater surprise to learn that I had become part of their lives, and they part of mine. It was something that was never mentioned in medical school and residency, and I began to realize that there was much that my training had not prepared me for. I didn't appreciate it at the time, but the important things about medicine and healing I would learn along my journey in medical practice and my patients would be my teachers.

While I always felt an important bond with all of my patients—a bond no doubt forged from professionalism and duty—some patients were more special than others. Some came to me through a listing in a telephone book, a few were sent by health insurance companies, and still others simply walked in off the street. Those that came on the recommendation of a colleague or a friend touched me deeply and I always seemed to work a little bit harder in order to honor the trust they had placed in me. Sometimes I knew that these patients would be special even before meeting them. Such was the case with Jack Hoff.

Early one morning, the turmoil of my office routine was interrupted by a rare telephone call that somehow managed to slip past the ruthless vigilance of the receptionist. I was taken aback by the voice of Herb Sefla on the receiver. I hadn't spoken to him since withdrawing from the oncology fellowship, and hearing his voice again filled me with a little apprehension. He told me that a close friend of his needed a doctor and asked if I would do him the favor of taking care of him. If I was surprised by the call, I was staggered by the request. There were many other doctors he could have called—most with far more experience than I—but he chose me. I felt a huge burden melt away. Things were alright between us. Perhaps this was where I was meant to be.

The very next morning, Jack Hoff, Dr. Sefla's boyhood friend, sat in one of my examination rooms. Obviously, his appointment had been scheduled long before Dr. Sefla called me and I suspected there was more to his presence than I was aware of. But there was little room for mystery and intrigue that day as the vibrancy and charm of this aging man filled the office so thoroughly. A mere glance at the man would bring a smile to one's face and memories of tender moments spent with fathers and grandfathers.

I too could only smile when I first entered the exam room. Upon seeing me he jumped to his feet and reached for my extended hand. The handshake apparently wasn't enough and quickly transformed into an embrace worthy of the best of friends.

"I'm so happy to meet you," he said. "I've heard so much about you and have waited so long, but some things are worth waiting for."

His spontaneity and ease surprised me a bit. There wasn't the slightest apprehension that I had grown accustomed to finding in patients meeting me for the first time. I too felt different than I usually did when meeting a new patient. It was as if we had known each other forever. It was like we were family.

"I knew we would be great friends," he went on, beaming. Growing thoughtful at my curious look, he added, "You've been my friend the minute Herb told me about you. And I am yours, you just don't know it yet, but that's okay. Heck, some of my best friends I haven't even met yet."

I could see him as Herb Sefla's friend. He was confident but unassuming and there was a distinct yet indescribable warmth about him that made you feel good just being around him. It would not be until later in my journey that I would recognize that warmth as healing, but I knew instantly that it was special. Like Herb, there was an air of wisdom about him but it was so much more. It seemed much too great to have been acquired during a mere seventy years of life. It seemed much too deep to have flowed from the experience of a single man, and it was much too vast to spring from the awareness of the human mind. While I knew little about Jack, I knew he was special and I knew that I liked him.

When we took our seats in the corner of the examination room, Jack motioned to a lady some thirty years his junior sitting next to him.

"I'd like to introduce Patty," he said.

"So this is your daughter?" I asked, lightly grasping her outstretched hand.

He tilted his head to one side and gazed at me with a quizzical look. "Patty is my wife," he said with a smile.

"I'm so sorry," I said, my face flushed in embarrassment.

"Don't be," Jack said, "her eternal youth just makes my life sing."

We didn't spend much time talking about Jack's health that first visit—something that my medical school teachers would have deemed unacceptable—but it seemed to be more important for us just to get to know each other. That understanding, I would soon come to learn, would be an essential ingredient of healing.

Jack was as mysterious as he was kind. An avid gardener with a strong love for nature, he seemed to know things about me that could only be learned by peering directly into my soul.

"He's a birder, honey." Jack excitedly said to his wife. "He found a saw-whet owl at the nature center. It's a fabulous bird, only about seven inches high and likes to sit in pine trees. I didn't even know we had them around here."

"How do you know he likes birds?" his wife asked him.

He looked at his wife in feigned disbelief. "Of course he likes birds," he said, "He's my friend."

"I didn't know that you liked birds," she replied.

"Of course I like birds," he responded, "I'm his friend."

Patty gave an exasperated sigh and shook her head slowly. "He gets like this," she said to me. "Take my advice, don't try to make sense of it. It will make you crazy."

Seldom have I enjoyed a visit with a patient more. As was often the case, the time I spent with them exceeded that which was allowed for on my schedule, but strangely I didn't care. Nothing instilled greater stress in me than running behind schedule, but on that day I never felt more relaxed. If I found it curious, my office staff was dumbfounded by it.

As Jack and Patty stood to leave, he mentioned he had to rush home to his garden and pepper his cabbage as it had rained the night before. She gave him a playful push toward the door and said, "Now I ask you. Have you ever heard anything as ridiculous as putting pepper on cabbage?"

'Yes," I said with some surprise. "My father used to do it. It's to prevent cabbage worms."

Jack gave his wife a triumphant *I told you so look* and with a wink whispered to me, "Who do you think told your dad?"

As he turned to leave, he paused for a moment and looked around at the walls of the small examination room. Growing serious he said, "You should really put some of your photographs up, Bill. There's wonderful energy captured in those images. You don't have to go to those places or see those things to experience that energy. You can bring part of it here to this place. It would help your patients."

I was going to ask Jack how he knew that photography was a

hobby of mine, but I probably wouldn't have believed, or understood, his answer. Suffice to say that Jack was one fascinating individual. Jack was much in my thoughts the rest of the day. I could picture him puttering in his garden, and as I watched, his image became that of my own father working in his garden. How much alike they were.

Home visited me that night. It was unusual of me to dream—or to at least remember the dreams by morning—but that night dreams came to me with uncommon brilliance. I was a boy again, home in my father's garden and possessed by the discovery of nature. The sweetness of a sun-ripened strawberry, the aroma of tomato leaves in the summer sun, and the velvet-like softness of a green bean's skin—my senses came of age in that garden and my soul was first touched by the energy of the natural world.

The dinner table was set with the delicacies of summer—steaming corn on the cob, tender carrots, mammoth baked potatoes, and succulent raspberries—all from the garden. They were mere overtures to the main event—the bacon, lettuce, and tomato sandwiches that sat in the middle of the table. We lived on them during the summer and never seemed to tire of their almost daily presence in our meals. It was part of the abundance that filled those years.

The following day was as hectic as the day before had been calm. Everything seemed to bring me stress—the overbooked schedule, paperwork at every turn, and the incessant ring of the telephone— but I couldn't rid my thoughts of those bacon, lettuce, and tomato sandwiches that had visited me the night before. I had forgotten about them and longed for their taste again. Just thinking about them seemed to make the day pass a bit easier and I vowed that I would stop by the store on my way home that night, seriously doubting, however, that I could find anything that came close to one of my father's tomatoes.

But it was not to be. A last-minute admission to the hospital, the laboratory's misplacing of urgently needed specimens, and a medical student seeking guidance on a research project all conspired to keep me at work much later than I had hoped. I couldn't bear the thoughts of the long line at the grocery store and instead drove straight home desperate for the peace I was sure to find there.

The sun was already setting as I pulled into my driveway and I sighed in resignation of the shortened evening that I would have at home. A large brown paper sack sat on my front porch and prevented my opening of the door. I was irritated by yet another obstacle that prevented my arrival home, as trivial and momentary as it was. I noticed that the sack was heavy as I carried it inside the house and placed in on the kitchen counter. I went through the mail and listened to my phone messages—entrenched rituals of my life—before satisfying my curiosity about the contents of the paper sack.

I gasped in shock when I opened that sack and peered inside. My hand trembled as I removed the loaf of bread, head of lettuce, jar of mayonnaise, package of bacon, and tomato from its interior. The tomato was huge and pristine. Not a single blemish marred its deep red skin. It was probably the largest tomato I had ever seen.

It wasn't long until tomato juice dripped from my chin, a tear or two collected in the corner of my eye, and a magnificent calm flowed over me. I was home again, refreshed by its innocence and reawakened to the exciting possibilities that I discovered there and had somehow forgotten about. I was home again and I knew without the slightest doubt that it was Jack Hoff who had taken me there.

It would be a couple of months before I would see Jack again and when he walked into my office for his next appointment, I calmly thanked him for the tomato and all the fixings. He didn't seem a bit surprised that I knew, nor did he feign ignorance of what I spoke of.

"Friends are always just a thought away," he said softly.

I saw Jack in the office every three months to monitor his high blood pressure. He would have come more often, but he was the healthiest retiree I had ever seen. Mostly he came to talk and there was never a visit when the day was not made better by his presence. He thrilled the office staff so completely that competition took place for the honor to usher him from the waiting room. But it wasn't necessary. Jack always made his rounds throughout the office on every visit just to chat with each and every employee. He knew them all by name and if they were not at work that day, they would receive a telephone call at home. Even a cranky old plumber working on a slow office drain left with a smile after meeting Jack. It was a strange paradox. Jack would go to the doctor's office to make everyone else feel better.

With every visit, Patty was at Jack's side. It was hard to picture one without the other. Her presence always reassured me. Jack was not the type of person to complain and I was always a bit suspicious on each office visit when he told me that it was impossible for him to feel better. I knew that Patty kept him honest.

It was much easier to be Jack's friend than it was to be his doctor. Talk of gardens, birds, and the wonderful people that he had met since his last visit always threatened to consume our time together before we had a chance to get down to business. He was a tough sell when it came to screening tests and health-maintenance procedures, convinced that it was the knowledge of an illness, not the actual illness itself, that influenced how one felt. He believed that people found what they thought about and looked for. When physicians, he insisted, spent too much time looking for illness rather than wellness, they were likely to find it.

After years of being amazed by Jack's seemingly endless supply of energy, I grew concerned one day that there might be trouble brewing on the horizon. While he insisted he was well and his physical examination seemed to agree with him, Jack just wasn't himself. Perhaps it was just the passage of time—Jack, was after all, halfway through his eighth decade of life—but such explanations didn't seem to fit Jack. Despite his stoicism, it was hard to deny that he had lost weight on each of his most recent office visits. My concern grew when I learned that he had reduced the size of his garden and I increased the frequency of his office visits so I could keep closer watch over him.

My concern grew to alarm one Sunday morning when Patty called me at home. Jack hadn't been out in his garden all week and he decided not to attend church that morning. It would be the first time they missed church since they had been married.

"Could he be depressed?" she wondered. "He sits for hours at a time doing nothing, but always has a smile on his face."

I couldn't imagine Jack being depressed, but then again I couldn't picture anything keeping him out of his garden. He refused my offer to meet them at the office, so I made my first house call. Patty was right—he was still smiling when I got there. It took less than a minute to make my diagnosis. Swollen feet and legs, engorged neck veins, and a crackling sound when listening to his lungs—Jack was in heart failure. He rebelled when I picked up the phone to call an ambulance, but just for a bit. This was one argument that I was going to win.

It didn't take long for the emergency room at the Teaching Hospital to confirm my diagnosis. Indeed, Jack had heart failure, and it was bad. His blood pressure was very low, his kidneys were failing, and the oxygen in his bloodstream was seriously reduced. Within an hour, he was in the cardiac catheterization laboratory. Within two hours, Jack was being wheeled into the operating room for emergency bypass surgery.

Open heart surgery is a challenge for anyone, but if you are a seventy-six-year-old man, the challenge can be one of survival. I was worried for the patient that had become my friend and spent the afternoon hovering near the operating room for news. Patty sat alone in the surgical waiting room quietly practicing the hopefulness that life with Jack had taught, but it was hard to remain cheerful around her when Jack's operation extended first one hour and then another beyond what we had expected. But the worry was a waste of energy—just as Jack would have admonished—and he made it through a difficult procedure without a single complication.

My first stop the following morning was the intensive care unit to check up on Jack. The chart and nursing notes brought a smile to my face. His vital signs, test results, and physical examination were those you would expect from a man half his age, but yet his nurses seemed worried.

"Maybe he's just disoriented," one nurse thought out loud," after all, he is getting up there in years."

"But he looks great," I objected as I looked in at Jack through the glass sliding door of his room. "Look at that smile on his face."

"Exactly," his nurse stated. "He's an old man who just had his chest cracked open and all he can do is smile. What the hell is he smiling about?"

Jack was delighted to see me, almost as much as I was to see him doing so well. I listened to his heart and lungs and noted with great satisfaction that the swelling in his legs was already better. Mostly though, we just talked. He looked amused when I told him that his nurses were worried that he looked too happy.

"Isn't that just like modern medicine," he said in mock disgust. "If patients aren't miserable, you guys think something is wrong. I smile when I'm happy. I've been visiting some wonderful places.

"Oh, by the way," he added almost as an afterthought. "You look just like your grandfather."

Perhaps his nurses were right. Maybe he was a little confused, but I didn't care. It was the Jack I had known for many years and even if I didn't always understand him, or even believe him much of the time, it did not diminish that special quality that could always be felt in his presence. It was good to have him back.

Less than a week after his surgery, Jack was home. While he was able to spend an hour or two in his garden each day, it was only to sit but not to work. His walks were much shorter and with a slower pace than had been his routine, and he lacked the energy to sit for hours at the barber shop trading stories with all who had become his friends. He used to hate taking naps but as the days passed, he gradually surrendered to their counsel, often with surprising frequency. If he noticed the changes, he never spoke of them. I never heard him complain.

Patty stopped by the office unexpectedly one morning, telling Jack she had to make a quick run to the grocery store. We were already overbooked with patients, but she needed to talk and so we did.

"He looks like an old man," she said with tears in her eyes. "It just happened. A few months ago he was fine."

"Well," I said softly, trying to choose my words carefully, "he is seventy-six, Patty. He's gone through surgery that would take a man half his age time to recover. You need to give him time."

"But he will get better?" she asked. "My father had major surgery and never was himself again before his death."

"Patty," I said with a deep breath, "the longer I do this and the more lives that touch mine, the less able I am to answer such questions. I haven't the wisdom. It's truly a journey and we never know what lies beyond the next rise in the road. But I do know this—the more we worry about what we might find beyond that next rise, the less able we are to see what surrounds us at the moment. If its great beauty that surrounds us, we may never see it. I don't know what is going to happen with Jack, but does it really matter? He's with us today.

"The differences in your ages—you must have considered the likelihood that he would reach the end of his life before you. Have you ever discussed it? Do you know what he would want if he was critically ill and couldn't speak for himself?"

"No, never. I guess we have been too caught up in the beauty to think about where the path may take us," she said with a soft smile.

"Then don't stop now, Patty," I said. "He's going to be an amazing man no matter where his journey takes him. To be able to share it with him is a precious gift."

There is a certain time of night after which a telephone call never brings good news. While I didn't look at the clock, there wasn't any doubt in my mind what kind of news the ringing telephone that woke me from a sound sleep was about to bring. I cringed when I heard Patty's voice on the line. Jack had passed out in the bathroom and she could not awaken him.

Jack was in a trauma room when I made it to the emergency department a half hour later. His blood count was very low and the doctors that huddled around him were worried about possible gastrointestinal bleeding. But his problems did not end there: he was again in heart failure, his blood pressure was critically low, his kidneys had stopped working. It was not a good place for an old man to be.

Jack was moved to the medical intensive care unit where a ventilator was placed at the ready, but the thought of using it made everyone feel uneasy. Jack stabilized somewhat over the remainder of the night. He certainly wasn't better, but we found some measure of satisfaction in knowing that his condition hadn't worsened any. As I stood outside Jack's room looking in, the duty that faced me weighed heavy on my soul. I was almost hoping he would be sleeping, but a weak smile spread across his face when he caught sight of me through the glass.

"How are you doing, Jack?" I asked, resting my hand on his.

His eyes grew misty as he looked at me. There was still the twinkle that I had come to know through the years. "Everyone's been so busy working on me and doing so much, but it wasn't until I saw you standing out there that I started to feel better."

"Jack," I said softly, "you're pretty sick but you're holding your own. I think you'll do just fine, but Jack, what if things get worse? Have you ever given any thought what you would like us to do if…"

"You've been worrying about this, haven't you?" Jack interrupted me. "I'm sorry for that. It isn't my time, Bill. I'm not sure how I know that, but I've never been more certain about anything. There are wondrous places still to explore and an abundance of time to do it in. I don't even have to leave this room to do it."

Jack placed the palm of his outstretched hand against my chest and said, "You do whatever feels right in here—no matter what your training tells you—and that's what will be best for me. That's what I want."

If I was hoping for the relief of a simple answer, I had forgotten who I was dealing with. But there would be no further guidance that morning. Exhausted by our brief conversation, Jack slipped off to sleep. Still, there was part of me that understood what he said to me and I found some irony in that realization. It would be one of the few times I had ever truly understood him.

The nurses—and a good number of my colleagues—were pressing for *do not resuscitate* and *comfort care only* orders, but they would not be written that day. Nor would they be written the day that followed, or the day after that. Oblivious of the statistics that foretold of old men in intensive care units, Jack showed improbable, albeit subtle, improvement over the following days. There was nothing subtle about his fourth day in the hospital, however. Every examination performed and every laboratory test drawn had dramatically improved from the ones done only hours earlier. The difference was as in night and day. The intensive care specialists could not explain his striking improvement, but somehow it seemed only fair—nobody could explain why Jack got so sick in the first place.

By his fifth day in the hospital, Jack was eating a regular diet, taking a few steps under the watchful eye of the physical therapist, and spending time sitting up in a chair. His talk of having visited a special place drove his nurses to distraction, convinced that he was suffering the aftermath of a brain that had been deprived of oxygen too long when he fell ill. They wanted me to call a psychiatrist.

Jack was sitting in a chair finishing his lunch when I walked into the room and sat down next to him. He looked great and all I could do was shake my head in disbelief, my smile spreading from ear to ear.

Jack put down his fork and with an atypically serious face, looked me in the eye and said, "I'm not nuts, doctor."

"Didn't think I knew, did you?" he said, his smile returning to his face. "That nurse out there has been measuring me for a straight jacket all morning." He had the look of a mischievous little boy when he told me that he had been having fun tormenting his young caregiver. "If they think you're crazy, then you might as well get some mileage out of it. I told her that I had just seen an elephant on roller skates and wearing a red dress in my room, but I was pretty sure it wasn't real. When she asked me what made me think it wasn't real, I told her that the elephant spoke to me in French and that everyone knows elephants only speak German."

He laughed so hard that I was afraid he was going to suffer a relapse. When he regained his composure, he asked, "Why is it that we call anything we don't understand *crazy*?"

Jack's face grew serious once more. "Would I have lived if they had made me *comfort care only*, Bill?" he asked.

I was visibly uncomfortable with the question and shifted uneasily in my chair.

"I thought so," Jack answered for me in a whisper. "Herb Sefla was right about you. He was so excited when he came to the house to tell me that he found a doctor for me. Herb had been taking care of me but it always made him feel uneasy. He thought I needed more. He knew that you were the one the day he met you. I just had to wait until you finished your training. Herb said it would be worth the wait. In my entire life, I've never known Herb to be wrong about anything."

"Jack," I said, flushing in embarrassment, "I just did what you told me to do."

Jack was having none of it. "You asked the question," he said simply. "You listened for the answer. The answer was important to you, even if you didn't understand it. Do you have any idea how special that is?"

I was desperate to change the subject. "There was nothing special here, Jack," I said, "except for the patient. But you know, Dr. Sefla couldn't have known that I was going into private practice. I didn't know myself until just a couple of months before I finished residency."

Jack raised his eyebrows and gave me a smile that I had seen many times before. "He knew," he said. "He knew before you knew. He was so disappointed when you wanted to go into oncology. He told me that you would make a fine oncologist but he just knew that the universe had something greater in store for you. My old friend was certainly right. I don't know where your journey is taking you, but I'm just thrilled to be sharing in part of it."

"Even if it means getting sick?" I teased.

"Especially by getting sick," Jack said in an unusually serious voice. "Until this year I had never been sick. I've been blessed with good health for which I have been profoundly grateful. But I've discovered that being sick is a blessing too."

He smiled at the confused look on my face. "Now remember," he said, "I'm not crazy."

Jack sat back in his chair, took a deep breath, and seemed to ponder just how to explain something that was obviously very important to him.

"There are places that are very special to me," Jack started slowly, "places where I feel good just because I am there, places where problems never seem as difficult, and places that seem a little closer to God than most. Some of these places are hard to get to or just far enough away that I don't make it there often enough; like the fabulous mountain peak in Colorado that I stumbled across one vacation as a young man, or the secluded little cove up at the lake. Some of those places are just outside my door—my backyard or my garden. But when I got sick, I couldn't make it even that far. And that's when I discovered it—the most special place that I have been."

"Where is this place, Jack?" I asked, intrigued by the almost reverent quality of his voice.

"Here," he said matter-of-factly.

"Here?" I asked, feeling a bit let down.

"Yes," he said, "right here."

"Now, Jack," I said as if I was addressing a young child, "do I have to go get that nurse and have her bring the jacket?"

It was like old times again when he laughed at my joke and it seemed just like yesterday when we had first met and got lost in talk of gardens and birds. It was hard to believe that he had been so very ill such a short time before.

"Here as in wherever you happen to be," he attempted to explain, "not just in this room, although I have grown quite fond of that IV pole," he said with a wink.

"When I was too weak to walk out to my garden, I was more frustrated than I had ever felt before. I could see it through the window but I could not be a part of it. I wondered if I would ever walk among my flowers again and felt an incredible sadness in every part of my body. I felt trapped, like being caught in a raging whirlpool with no way to escape. Whenever I had felt sad before, a walk in my garden was all it took to start feeling better again. But I couldn't do that, which made me feel even worse.

"But something happened in midst of that whirlpool. Every time an image of my garden swirled by in my thoughts, I could see it a bit clearer and hold on to it a little longer. Soon I could feel the softness of grass beneath my feet and the gentle breeze against my face. The waters grew calm and my thoughts became real. I was once again standing in my garden, savoring the tenderness and fragrance of rose petals and the calm that I feared had eluded me forever.

"It was the most amazing discovery. All I had to do was grow quiet and think about those special places and they were brought to me, or I to them. With it came the peace and understanding that I had always felt there. The realization that I was in fact at those special places—without ever leaving my chair—was as astonishing as it was empowering. I could go to places where there were answers to any question, wisdom for any situation, and peace for any problem—in the instant of a thought.

"I've visited so many wonderful places since getting sick and even while being here in the hospital. Surely, there have been times when you have felt so good that all you can do is smile. That's the way it's been with me."

I had entered Jack's room with the intention of spending time with a friend and perhaps honor the confused thoughts of an old man, but the longer I sat there the more intrigued I became with him and his unusual story. It was impossible to dismiss him, even if I didn't truly understand him. I felt strangely aware of the magical teachers that had blessed my career—from the accident scene as a paramedic to the bedside of a dying man as a young physician—that I had never understood.

"So you are telling me that the special place is here," I said, "because you can make any room or any place special?"

"To a point," Jack said after pausing for a moment of thought, "but it goes deeper than that. The *here* refers more to time than it does a place. *Here* is *right now* or *the present moment*. The place, well it's actually us. I've always been taught that there is a place within us that connects us with the universe, and at times I've had awareness of it—flashes of understanding, moments filled with spine-tingling awe, and somehow just knowing that I was part of something great—

but it wasn't until being taken there very recently that I touched the miraculous. My entire life has been simply wonderful, but I've always had the vague feeling that I was looking for something. There is no doubt in my mind that I've found it.

"We all have something or somebody that can take us to this place. Maybe for you it's a titmouse—for me it's a butterfly. I've always been fascinated by those wondrous wisps of life. It's how I started gardening. I'd plant anything that would attract butterflies. Now I realize that they helped me create that wonderful piece of heaven. Now when I'm quiet I can picture a favorite place—my garden or perhaps the lake—and watch the butterfly. It seems to float on nothing more than spirit and as I concentrate on it, I slip deep into the stillness of my being and find the most marvelous place waiting for me. When we learn to quiet all the noise in our lives and actually experience the present moment, we can discover that special place within us. We can go there whenever and wherever we choose. I've seen the most incredible sights and met the most remarkable souls while there. It is our link with every life that has ever lived and with every atom in the universe. Imagine what healing secrets you could bring back from such a place. But it's a place that you won't find unless you look for it, or allow yourself to be taken there."

As Jack spoke, he reached for the piece of cherry pie that remained on his lunch tray. I watched in startled fascination as he rotated the pie so that the crust was facing him before picking up his fork to eat. I had only seen two others eat pie crust first like that: my father and his brother. It was something that their father had taught them, or perhaps it was something that the boys had taught their father. Pie was a rare treat in the farmhouse in which they were raised during the Depression. While there was nothing that their mother wouldn't do for them, the lady couldn't bake pie crust to save her soul. It was law—if the crust went uneaten, there would be no more pies made. So the men of the house learned to eat the crust first and save the best part of the pie for last.

Jack noticed the strange way that I looked at him. Gesturing at the pie with his fork—and with what I was certain was a twinkle in his eye—he said, "The crust is so bad here that I eat it first and save the best part for last."

Was it a coincidence or did he somehow know? It was a question that disturbed my thoughts for the rest of the day and most of the sleepless nights that followed. Perhaps the nurses were right and Jack was a little crazy, but his observation was also correct—we tend to view those who we do not understand as crazy. The nurses had praised the way I listened to Jack and humored the musings of an old man, but it was more than gracious listening that had kept me at his side. Whether I understood him or not, the time that I spent with Jack always left me feeling at peace and comfortable with the realization that I had so much more to learn. Somehow, the prospect excited me.

Jack was right about something else. It was not his time. Two days later, he left the hospital and returned to his garden and the wonders that I was certain he would find there. It always made me feel good to see a patient leave the hospital, but with Jack, it was particularly sweet. There were still wondrous places for him to explore and I was looking forward to hearing about them.

I felt unusually rested when I returned home that night. I paused on the porch after retrieving the mail and looked around my small yard with eyes that seemed to see it differently than before. The evening was far too pleasant to go inside so I sat down on the steps to enjoy it while I thumbed through the mail. An envelope with my brother's handwriting made me smile and I opened it immediately. A note and photograph were inside. It was a short note telling of a discovery in an old chest in my parents' attic and asking if I ever wondered what I was going to like when I got older. The photograph was yellowed with age and on the back was written my grandfather's name and the year 1952. I never knew my grandfather—he died when I was very young—and I never recalled ever having seen a picture of him. As I turned over the photograph, my curiosity turned to astonishment. Pictured leaning against a wonderfully old automobile was a tall and slender man. It was the same image, albeit some years older, that peered out at me from the bathroom mirror every morning. The recognition came with the realization that I too had wondrous places to explore.

The titmouse's call brought my thoughts back from the memories of Herb Sefla and Jack Hoff to the stillness of Demazie Hollow. I couldn't help but wonder if it was the same bird that had led me to this place, much like the butterflies that helped Jack discover his garden. It seemed appropriate that Jack would visit me here. It was only after coming here that I started to understand much of what we had talked about. Only after our journeys took separate paths did my friend and patient become my teacher. Perhaps that is what made this place so special. Here the student became ready.

CHAPTER 5

Healing Is but a Thought Away

*You are today where your thoughts have brought you; you
will be tomorrow where your thoughts take you.*

JAMES ALLEN

I sat watching the old lady in the frayed and faded pink dress, which was held together by strategically placed gold safety pins. She had a pride about her as she sat erect in the waiting room chair. It was as if she was wearing her Sunday best and I was reasonably certain that she was.

I was sure it was the same woman I had seen picking blackberries along the gravel road leading to Demazie Hollow. It had been an unusually bountiful crop and her dented bucket overflowed with succulent fruit. Her face bore a broad grin—much like that of a child's when exploring the wonders contained within the bakery's glass display case—the same face that smiled at me when I walked through the waiting room of the free clinic. The two missing front teeth made it a difficult smile to forget.

It was appropriate that she was here as the clinic sprouted from the seeds that I found in Demazie Hollow many years earlier and grew in the nourishment of the energy that touched me there. Jack Hoff—my old friend and teacher—was right; we can return to special places with a thought and take the wisdom that we find there with us in the energy of our soul, and share it with others.

The stunning beauty that I found in Appalachia could not hide the need that lived in meager shelters, cut tobacco in the summer, and hunted the woods and fields in the fall. It was all part of what made it special, as was the opportunity to serve. The free clinic was much more than a place to give, for no matter how great the number of patients or the complexity of the problems that we cared for, at the end of the day we left with much more than we had given. It was all part of the energy that flowed from a special place.

I was atypically early to clinic that day and was surprised to find that the old lady had been waiting for many hours. She didn't have a car—never learned how to drive for that matter—and caught a ride into town with a man that traveled to the city very early every morning. She didn't know how she was to get home but she showed little concern. Her needs always seemed to be met in just the right way and at just the right time. I thought about seeing her early so that she would not have to wait any longer but something urged me not to. It would be a shame to deprive the medical residents the opportunity to care for someone whom I was certain was going to be a very special person.

It did not take long for the intern and senior resident to arrive. They had shared a ride from the city and judging from their smiles, it had been a good trip. It was always good to see a resident smile as happiness seemed a rare thing during the training years. I recognized the first-year resident as she rushed through the door. It was Samantha and she was beyond happy. She was positively ecstatic.

"We just saw a roadrunner!" she shouted excitedly.

"I don't think so," I said, trying to stifle a chuckle. "The roadrunner is a desert bird. You see them out west and in Texas."

"No, I'm sure it was a roadrunner," Sam insisted. "It was black, larger than a chicken, and had a long neck and tail. And boy did it run fast across the road."

"You saw a turkey," I suggested.

"Turkeys are white," replied a confused-looking Sam. "I've been to a turkey farm back home."

"Domestic turkeys are white," I said, losing my battle to keep a straight face. "We have the real thing here, and yes, they are wonderful birds. You should see them in the spring when the males display their fanned tails."

A strange cackling sound silenced our conversation and drew our attention to the waiting room. The old lady in the pink dress was leaning forward and her shoulders heaved up and down as she desperately tried to silence her laughter. She grew visibly embarrassed when she noticed us looking at her and hid her face in her hands.

"Well," Sam said with a smile, "at least I can bring humor into people's lives."

While only a few months had passed since I first met Sam, the changes were hard to miss, even for a casual observer. There was a confidence about her. She had made the transition from student to doctor and it was a thrill to watch her work. While the fear that I once saw in her eyes was gone, something had taken its place. It was hidden well behind the sparkle of her personality and the gleam of discovery and mastery, but it was there. It was a touch of sadness, one that I had often seen in other young doctors through the years but never paid much attention to.

Sam disappeared behind the examination room door with the old lady from the hills. She did not know it then, but she would be forever changed when she emerged from that room. The exam room walls were paper-thin and it was not difficult to hear what was being said from my seat on the other side. There was talk of turkeys and other game birds that blessed Appalachia—ruffed grouse, quail, and on rare occasions, a pheasant—and there was laughter that perhaps a roadrunner or two might be seen. There was talk of lush green hills, winding country roads, crystal clear streams, and there was talk of home.

It seemed far too long to Sam since she had been home and the drive through the country took her back to the small town were life seemed simple and calm. While she had never given it much thought previously, the dreams that led her to medicine had started in that place and she felt a strange pull to return one day with the fortunes gleaned from her journey to the big city. Grams—the old lady had known no other name for such a long time—had never traveled far from her wooded hills. She was born there, raised a family there, and no doubt would move on there. It was home and she was eager to share.

She spoke of goldenrod, red clover, and blazing star—pigments that helped paint the late summer tapestry she savored every day on her walks. She talked about trees and which would be the first to lose its leaves in the fall, show the greatest color, and make the best firewood. She spoke of wild animals that shared her home—the deer that grazed nearby, the red fox that always sat in the morning sun not far from her door, and of the coyotes that sang her to sleep each night. It was home of which she was proud and grateful.

Grams was the keeper of secrets, secrets passed on by her grandmother who had inherited them from her grandmother. They were precious secrets and in the tradition of her family, she shared them with all in need. There was snakeroot for rheumatism, tulip tree bark for indigestion, and colt's foot for cough. She would gather goldenseal to treat eye infection and dig black cohosh to help with the time of life. While she had helped countless through the years, her cures and remedies didn't always work well when she applied them on herself. She was grateful it wasn't the other way around.

She had heard about the doctors that traveled from the city, and while she was reluctant to go and embarrassed that she could not treat herself, perhaps the outsiders would be able to help her. She felt rather guilty at taking the doctors' time for such a simple problem when there were so many others with far greater need, but it just wasn't for herself. Many depended on the preserves and canned goods that she put up and the hand pain and stiffness was making the task difficult. It would be winter soon and she had much work yet to do. Maybe the doctors could help her just a little. She could live with the pain as long as she was able to work.

It would be an hour before Sam left Grams in the examination room. She had a curious look of fascinated excitement about her when she sat down in the chair across from me. "What an incredible lady," she said. "I'm sorry I took so long. I just couldn't leave."

Sam grew quiet and sat back in her chair with a faraway look about her. I thought she was collecting her thoughts before telling me about her patient, but when several minutes had passed in silence, I nudged her back to the present moment.

"Sorry," she said with a start at the sound of her name. "I was thinking about a patient I saw this morning. I've seen Mr. Woodmont—that's his name—a couple of times now and it never takes him more than a minute or two to tell me how poor he is. I've always felt sorry for him. He gets county assistance and has a medical card. Every time I write him a prescription, he reminds me how unfair it is that he has to pay two dollars for every medication he gets filled. The county expects him to work a few hours each week for his check but this morning he wanted a statement that he was too ill to work. He's forty-two years old and his only problem is back pain."

"And this has what to do with the patient you just saw?" I asked gently.

"Sorry," she said again, looking rather uncomfortable. "It's just that Grams is poor too, but I don't think she knows. In fact, I think she considers herself well off. I asked her about her income and she told me that she gets a check for $446 every month in survivor benefits after her husband was killed while working at some power plant thirty years ago. She was embarrassed to tell me about the check, not because it is so small, but because it is so much more than her neighbors have.

"Four hundred and forty-six dollars a month! That wouldn't make my car payment. It's almost like there are two types of poverty. Those who know they are poor and live in scarcity and those—like Grams—who don't view themselves as poor and live in abundance."

"Wow," I said, "that's some powerful insight, Sam. So what's wrong with Grams?"

"It's pretty classic osteoarthritis," she said. "She has it pretty bad in her hands and that's what is having the biggest impact on the quality of her life."

As we were discussing Grams, one of the clinic staff placed a small paper bag and some change on the desk in front of Sam. "This is what you wanted from the drug store," she said.

"What are you going to do for Grams?" I asked.

"I was going to send her out with some samples of NSAIDs," Sam replied, "but I think capsaicin cream would help her a lot and would be a better fit with her holistic side."

"That's an excellent idea," I said, "but it doesn't sound like she can afford capsaicin cream. It's over-the-counter but is rather pricey."

Seeing the sheepish grin on Sam's face, I added, "Or is that what's in the bag?"

"I told her we had some free samples," Sam said a bit apologetically, "but I don't see why she needs to know where it really came from. I don't think she would take it otherwise and I really believe it will help her."

I glanced at the nurse who was hovering nearby, curious to learn the reason for the unusual trip to the corner drug store. I thought I could see a tear in the corner of her eye. If you looked closely, you probably would have been able to see a tear in the corner of my eye as well. Even Sam's eyes looked a little different. Somehow, they seemed a little less sad than they had just an hour before.

The remainder of the afternoon was a blur of activity. We had fallen behind while seeing Grams, but nobody seemed to mind. The full waiting room was the definition of patience—everyone knew there would be time enough for them when it was their turn. I would have been stressed beyond belief if in my office back in the city, but even my angst at running late was calmed by the energy of the country. There was never a scarcity of time here.

Everyone who visited the clinic was poor—it was, after all, a free clinic—but I couldn't help but reflect upon Sam's hypothesis that there were two types of poverty. The county that the clinic served was among the poorest in the state. There were few jobs for those who wanted to work and what jobs were available could seldom provide much of a wage. For many, days were spent in front of the television where images of abundance made scarcity's sting a bit more obvious. For others, talk radio suggested who was to blame for their misfortune. Drug abuse thrived and substances that promised escape were never far away. It was a cauldron of circumstance and vulnerability from which victims arose.

Tabetha Sloan was a victim. Months earlier, the twenty-two-year-old single mother had come to the clinic requesting an MRI for back pain that wouldn't go away. It was a study that she couldn't afford and one that her symptoms and examination did not warrant, but she was adamant. The man she talked to on the telephone told her that he could help her if she had an MRI. She saw his phone number on a television commercial that promised money to all who had been injured. Tabetha had slipped on eggs at the local grocery store, and while she was the one that had dropped the eggs, the man on the phone assured her that the store was at fault for having a floor that could get slippery.

It is hard for victims to find healing. When the source of unhappiness lies outside of themselves, so too must be sought the answers. Happiness is seldom found there. The medication Tabetha received at the clinic on her first visit didn't bring her happiness and neither did that received on the second and third visits. She didn't do any of the exercises that they recommended; movement just made her back hurt more. But she did find doctors and nurses that seemed willing to listen—for as long as she needed to talk—and somewhere during the process she discovered that she wasn't alone and perhaps life wasn't as bleak as those television commercials made it seem. She turned off the television, started to take long walks, and spent much of the day helping the many elderly in the apartment complex where she lived. She liked helping others—it made her feel good—and in sharing in the lives of others, she couldn't help but notice how much she had to be grateful for.

Tabetha wasn't complaining of back pain the day Sam saw her in the clinic. She had a form that needed to be completed by a physician before she could become a home health aid. The thought came to her during one of her walks. She never imagined she could get paid for doing something she enjoyed. The company she was going to work for would send her to school to become a medical assistant. Maybe she would even become a nurse someday. The thought excited her thoroughly—as completely as thoughts of pain and scarcity had once filled her with unhappiness—and it dawned on her that she had control over how she felt.

Sam looked a little disappointed when our last patient left the clinic. Something about her was different. Somewhere amidst the emphysema, diabetes, and loneliness that filled our afternoon, Sam had changed. It was subtle, but it was clearly there. I could see it in her smile, her voice, and in those eyes. The sadness that I thought I had seen earlier was gone. Perhaps I had imagined it. She stood gazing out the window as I wrote my final chart note and would occasionally look back at me as if to make certain I was still there.

"Samantha," I said softly. "You look like you have something on your mind."

"No," she said in an almost sad voice, "I'm just happy."

"You don't sound happy, Sam," I replied.

"It worries me a bit," she said softly.

"Sure," I said in a dry voice, "I always worry when I feel happy."

She smiled at my attempted sarcasm and sat down in a chair next to me. "I don't think I have ever felt happier," she said wistfully, "and I'm worried it won't last when I go back."

She studied the confused look on my face and continued, "I've wanted to be a doctor for as long as I can remember. I've even pictured myself in a small town—something like this one. But the past couple of months I've been worried that I made a huge mistake. After all the years in college and medical school—now that I made it—I haven't been so sure I want to be a doctor.

"Once the terror of my first month wore off, I kept waiting for those good feelings that I dreamed about for so long, but they never came. Nobody looks happy in this business—nurses, social workers, pharmacists, and even the other residents—everyone looks beaten down. The attendings have been the hardest to watch. You guys are in the hospital at all hours of the day and night and you always look sad. If it happens to our mentors, what chance do we have?"

I noticed a tear in Sam's eye and a catch in her voice as she continued. "So I've been worried that I made a mistake; that after all these years of work, I wasn't going to find my dream—until today. This is what I've been looking for. This is what I've always thought medicine was about. This is what I've wanted to do and today I discovered that it was possible. I believe that I actually helped people today; that I might have made a small difference. I've never been sure of that feeling before.

"When I realized that it's time to be heading back to the city, I found myself starting to worry again because I'm not so sure that I want to go back; that this wonderful feeling can't survive at the hospital. But you know what? It doesn't matter. Today has happened and no matter what tomorrow might bring, nothing can change what I experienced here."

Sam grew still for a moment and smiled. It was perhaps the most radiant smile I had ever seen. "If I should die tomorrow," she said with a reverence in her voice, "I shall do so knowing I have lived my dream."

I'm not sure how long we sat together in silence—a few seconds or maybe many minutes—as time stood motionless. The hum from the refrigerator in the corner was the only sound to break the quiet and even that seemed unusually muted, perhaps in respect of the moment. It was a profoundly special moment—one of many that had hallowed a life of practice and of teaching—and I wondered how many others had slipped away unnoticed into the illusion of haste and confusion that had filled my days. It was an awareness that I would come to treasure as every patient and student would bring the potential of extraordinary discovery and uncommon contentment. It made my skin tingle with excitement.

"You'll feel this at home, Sam," I said reassuringly. "The happiness is not here. It's not in these patients. The happiness is in you. It's in all of us but can remain hidden for much of our lives. It's like the spring wildflowers that I love so much. Every winter I forget just where they grow but with the warmth and light of spring, they sprout up from hidden roots. There is an energy here to be sure—an energy that has awakened something special within you, something that has always been there, and something that you will not long forget. You can take this energy wherever you go. When the needs of others seem so much greater than your capacity to give, all you have to do is think about today—the beauty of the countryside, the people, and the opportunity you have had to serve—and the answers will be clear to you and the feeling that fills you so completely now will return.

It's all just a thought away.

"Maybe healing is nothing more than changing the energy that surrounds us—the energy of our thoughts, our environment, and what we do—to a higher and more nurturing level. Look at Tabetha. When she changed what she thought about, what she surrounded herself with, and how she spent her time, not only did her back pain disappear, but she discovered new potential in life. But maybe the biggest impact is on us. Today she was our teacher. She taught us about healing.

"Just because we are doctors doesn't mean healing is for someone else. You say that yesterday you felt sad and worried that you misspent your life, but today you found happiness and the certainty of purpose. Can there be any better definition of healing than that? It can be ours for a thought."

A soft tapping drew our attention to the office door. There, a middle-aged woman stood holding a huge zucchini in rough, weathered hands. "Mrs. Stoker," I said in surprise, "did we forget you? I'm so sorry. I didn't know you had an appointment."

"Oh, I'm not here to be seen, doctor," she said. "I stopped by to leave this for you."

Turning to Sam, she said, "He just loves zucchini and I've been nursing this one for weeks. It's been so dry that it's needed watering every day."

She beamed when I told her it was the finest zucchini I had ever seen. Embarrassment clouded her face when I thanked her for her generosity and she left as quickly and as quietly as she had come.

"You must really like zucchini," Sam said with an amused look.

"Actually," I sighed. "I loath zucchini."

"Then why?" Sam asked with a laugh.

"Because it's all she has," I said softly, "and it gives her the opportunity to give. And it gives me the opportunity to feel grateful. You see, she is one of my teachers."

CHAPTER 6

It's Just Chaos Here

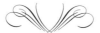

In all chaos there is a cosmos, in all disorder a secret order.

CARL JUNG

*If we could read the secret history of our enemies, we would find in
each person's life sorrow and suffering enough to disarm all hostility.*

HENRY WADSWORTH LONGFELLOW

Demazie Hollow was everything that the practice of medicine
had not been to me. Once the terror of those first years of
practice had melted into the comfort of routine, the predictability of
common diseases that occurred commonly had brought confidence
to my day, and after struggling with the arrogance that invariably
accompanies the mastery of facts, I discovered the penetrating satisfaction that I had always hoped medicine would bring me. A life
consumed with work that yielded little time for family and friends
seemed a small price to pay for the opportunity to dance in one's own
dream. I had found what I had looked for. I had looked for what I
had known about. I was unprepared for the knowledge that there
was more, but grateful for the teachers that would help me find it.

I had grown accustomed to the frenetic pace of medicine. The majority of my day was spent always late for something. Accomplishing only a single task in a given moment seemed a tragic waste of energy. The not-yet-read journal sitting on my desk would invariably contain the answers that might cure my next patient. I could identify the illnesses born of stress in my executive patients but was oblivious to the realization that their symptoms had become a part of my own life.

Medicine was a world of scarcity. Demazie hollow was one of abundance. The distinction took me by surprise even on my first visit. There was endless calm in the woods and something wonderful to ponder behind every tree that stretched as far as the eye could see. My office schedule was filled daily not with an abundance of illness, but with a scarcity of health. It was a perception of lack that was addressed in kind. Obviously, the patient needed more—more tests, more specialists, and more medications.

There was a curious anxiety that accompanied me on my early visits to the woods. Surely, I should be doing something better with my time—telephone calls to return, reading to catch up on, or the stack of paperwork that cluttered my desk. The calmness I felt there was distracting at first. The challenging diagnoses that typically filled my thoughts when away from the office were difficult to focus upon. The incessant chatter within my mind was strangely quiet and I felt somewhat lost without the noise. The many that always surrounded me were gone—it was only me and I was almost certain I could hear the woods speaking.

Ironically, I was deeply entrenched in the world of medicine when I first appreciated the incredible power of Demazie Hollow. There had been two hospital admissions the previous night but I only had time to see one of them before making it to the office—and even then I was considerably late. The waiting room was packed with patients as I walked through feeling immensely self-conscious amidst the countless stares. The receptionist was engaged in a heated dispute with an older lady that stood at the counter insisting that she had an appointment and even had the appointment card that was mailed to her to prove it. Seven telephone messages already waited on my desk, four of which were considered urgent and the laboratory had called to inform us that a pap smear we had performed the week before revealed cervical cancer.

Half of our lunch period was gone by the time I finished seeing my last patient of the morning and I still had to make it to the hospital before the afternoon session started. The staff looked exhausted and my desk looked like a bomb had gone off on it.

"What did you do yesterday?" my nurse Erin asked.

"Nothing special," I answered. "I did some housework and went to the woods. Why do you ask?"

"Because you're smiling," she said.

"I always smile," I replied.

"True," she said, "but now you look like you mean it."

"What's that supposed to mean?" I laughed.

"Didn't we have a patient that always used to say that he smiled because he was happy?" she asked.

"What of it?" I asked, feeling a bit interrogated.

"Do you feel happy?" she pressed. "I mean on a day like this? You're not going to have time for lunch; you still have calls to return, and we have a full schedule this afternoon for which you will never make it back on time for. Running behind schedule always makes you crazy. What gives?"

"I guess I do feel happy," I mused. "I'm amazed how much better Mrs. Smith felt just by talking and I don't care what the surgeon says, Mr. Harrold is doing great."

"You know," Erin said in her best motherly voice, "you looked the same way a couple of weeks ago after you had been to the woods. Maybe there is a message here."

Erin was right. I did feel better than I normally did after seeing patients, even when the schedule ran smoothly. I'm not sure I would have noticed had she not said something. I sat quietly in my office—oblivious to the concern that I was still running late—and pondered what I was feeling. The calm I felt in the woods—I could feel a part of it now. That strange feeling of awe—it was there as well.

There are other places that I have come to know as special, but Demazie Hollow is unique among them. With every visit, a part of it leaves with me. Jack Hoff knew of such things. He pondered the energy that could be found there and what magic it might work in a healer's life. Indeed, there was a healing energy in the hollow—stress, anger, and negative emotion simply can't survive there—but I was far from the first to recognize it. Shawnee shamans roamed these woods long ago and mastered its secrets. The old lady who lives on a nearby ridge knows every plant and herb that grows here and has practiced healing for three generations. The country preacher speaks of souls that have been healed here.

At times, the practice of medicine can be a daunting task with patients seeking answers that we do not know and wisdom that we do not have. For matters of cure, I turn to the journals that line my walls, the best technology that medicine has to offer, and the brightest minds that a teaching hospital can attract. When I need to know about healing, it is not uncommon to find me in the woods.

More often than not, turmoil seems to define my days in medicine. Often, I am amazed that we are able to care for the illness that seeks us out amid the overbooked schedules, the micromanagement of insurance carriers, and the maze of bureaucracy that the office staff face each day, but somehow we do. Our ability to heal is altogether a different question, one that I contemplated from the large rock beneath the red oak in Demazie Hollow. I was intrigued with the flight of a butterfly and I couldn't help but think of how excited it would have made Jack Hoff. It was a spicebush swallowtail and occasional bursts of iridescent colors would flash from its wings as it moved through the filtered sunlight of the woods. It would fly in high spiraling circles before coming to a momentary rest on a Joe-Pye weed and then move haphazardly to a nearby tall ironweed. In moments, it would again float erratically until coming to rest once again on the flowering domes of the Joe-Pye weed. It was such a chaotic flight that it reminded me of the disorder I had left behind at the office and which would invariably be waiting for my return on Monday morning.

Chaos was not a stranger to medicine. While it seemed to be everywhere, there was no place where it was more institutionalized than the VA hospital. While it had been many years since I first walked through its doors as an attending physician, I still felt a twinge of apprehension when facing a new team for the first time. It could be a difficult place but the patients were unlike any others and I enjoyed being there. The VA hospital was situated at the foot of a steep hill, the top of which sat the Teaching Hospital. I paused for a moment along the walk from my office at the Teaching Hospital to the VA hospital where my new team would soon meet.

I shuddered when I looked down from the top of the hill. It

was bedlam. While barely seven o'clock in the morning, the air was filled with horns, the pounding and clanging of equipment, and with shouts. Scores of cars continuously circled the parking lots in a vain search for spots to park, which did not exist. Ambulances lined up and down the road, waiting for their turn to unload. It was bedlam. I had seen it before, but yet there was something different.

A long series of cement steps made the descent down the hill possible. There had always been a small sign at the midway point announcing the transition between Teaching Hospital property and that of the VA. The sign that stood there now was immense. It proclaimed entry onto federal property and in bold block letters listed the many demands expected of all who entered. It did not speak of welcome.

Freshly poured cement columns rose vertically from each side of the walkway and piles of bricks, sand, and fencing material were scattered about. It struck me as curious. Why would a VA hospital need a fence? Was it to keep something in or a barrier to those who sought to enter?

The VA was in full construction mode and the grounds were a hive of activity. From a parking lot that once served patients grew the cement, brick, and motor of a hospital addition. It had been there six months earlier when I last walked by and three months before that. Despite the small army of men wearing hardhats milling about and those in suits with clipboards that conspicuously watched them, it had changed little. I was almost certain that those four men had been working on that same door six months earlier.

The brand new condos that sat across the street from the VA hospital, on the other hand, they hadn't been there six months earlier. Where old and dilapidated houses once stood, a miracle had taken place. They seemed purposefully placed to stand in contrast with what was possible at the VA.

The door—like all the windows on the new structure—was darkly tinted. It was impossible to see inside and I wondered if it was a cosmetic choice or one of substance. The lack of transparency almost seemed symbolic of the VA.

The construction of the addition to the hospital necessitated the creation of a new entrance, but the reorganized traffic pattern was less forgiving than its predecessor. Cars, ambulances, wheelchairs, and walkers all competed for the same handicap area. The congestion was formidable and rivaled the confusion of the morning commute on the expressway.

There were two doors entering the hospital—a revolving door like those seen at large airports, and a smaller, traditional door. A guard stood outside the traditional door and directed those who tried to pass to use the revolving one. The revolving door was huge and could accommodate ten or more people at a time. It moved painfully slow and quickly filled to capacity, often including men in wheelchairs, using walkers, or limping with canes. It was a strange sight—a tightly packed group advancing slowly one small step at a time—one that probably would have made me laugh had it not been happening to me. As we inched forward, I wondered about the door's purpose—to save energy or exert control?

The door opened into the spacious lobby through which I had walked many times, weaving through and around countless men. The faces all looked younger to me but the eyes were the same—some looked sad, others frustrated, and still others resigned. They all seemed to have a story to tell. It was the eyes of the women though that I noticed the most. Clutching the hands of husbands, fathers, and brothers, they shared a special journey. The lobby was choked with humanity.

In the time it took to walk from the revolving door to the elevators, my pager sounded three times. I was irritated when I saw that same telephone number on the pager's display three consecutive times and with the impatience of the person that was waiting there. Locating a house phone, I dialed the strange number. It was the hospital operator.

"I have the chief of staff holding on an outside line, doctor," the anxious voice told me. "He's upset and he doesn't like to be kept waiting."

In a matter of seconds, a new voice came on the line. It was a loud and angry-sounding voice. "This is Dr. Axforth," the male voice said. "I don't know you but you obviously know that I'm chief of staff. One of your patients, a Ronnie Smitt, called me at eleven last night to complain about the bad care that you are giving him. The poor guy is in pain and you are ignoring him. This is despicable and I just won't tolerate it in my hospital."

"I'm sorry to hear about this," I said. "I'm just coming on service but I will investigate this right away and get back with you."

"No, no, no," he snapped. "It's already been investigated. He called me so it's true. I already told him that you were at fault and that you would apologize first thing this morning. After you do that you are going to give this man whatever he wants for pain and as often as he wants it."

"We will certainly see him on rounds along with all of the other patients this morning, Dr. Axforth," I responded in measured words, trying hard to keep my composure. "I'll make sure that he gets the same good care that all of our patients receive."

Instead of a reply, I heard a loud click and then silence. It was a delightful silence and I was reluctant to hang up the phone and go find my team. It appeared that it was going to be an interesting month. If I had thought I had seen bedlam looking down at the VA hospital from the top of the hill, the view up close and personal was no better. It was a horrible way for residents to start a ward month—being on call the very first day. But that was the way my team was introduced to the VA hospital. They had been up all night admitting new patients while struggling to learn about those that they inherited from the previous team. The last thing that they wanted to do was meet a new attending physician and sit though two hours of rounds—they had too much work to do.

As a brand new second-year resident, it was Bruce Singleton's first month as a team leader and he was obviously nervous. He had a right to be. The VA was a tough place for senior residents. At night, they were the most experienced medicine doctors in the hospital and their pagers went off accordingly. He had planned for this month a long time and wanted things to be perfect. But this was the VA and perfection was an elusive thing.

I had seen the look before. He had intended to impress his new attending on the first morning rounds, but ambition and hard work was no match for the reality of the VA hospital. Morning labs not drawn, medication orders not processed, vital signs not obtained, and patients not being transported for scheduled tests—nothing went according to plan or how one would expect a hospital to function. I had seen that look of defeat and surrender on residents' faces many times at the VA, but that morning I thought I could see some fear in those eyes.

It was perhaps the most painful rounds I had ever endured.

Patient presentations—typically thorough, well thought out, and polished to an exceptional shine—were simply horrible. Patient histories were either incomplete or entirely lacking, physical examinations seemed cursory, and the assessments left me wondering whether the young doctors adequately knew their patients. It was a thought that had never crossed my mind in the many years I had attended at the VA and the Teaching Hospital. I felt a panic grow deep inside—perhaps Dr. Axforth was right and there was a serious problem on my team.

I was too bewildered speak; my thoughts trapped somewhere between anger and shock. As I looked from face to face in that conference room, I could almost see myself sitting there so many years before as an attending physician ranted and raved about the quality of his team's work. I felt embarrassed by the memory, not because of its substance but by how close I had come to repeating history.

The conference room where we gathered for rounds each morning did nothing to help me find calm before addressing my team. The lights—controlled by an electronic apparatus at the door—would spontaneously turn off then back on again. It was not a new problem and it had been baffling the maintenance department for many years, or perhaps they simply grew weary of trying. The light demons were unusually active that morning, exercising their control every two or three minutes. They seemed to work in concert with the inexorable force that enticed an almost continuous din from pagers and telephones. The construction work below rattled the conference room windows and one wondered what an earthquake must be like.

"We need to do better than this," I told my team softly. "It would appear that either we do not know what is wrong with our patients and how to take care of them, or we have failed in communicating that. I don't believe the former for an instant, so we are going to work on letting others know what great doctors you are. Look, I'm concerned first and foremost that our patients get the best care we can provide to them, but presentations and write-ups are important too. In medical education, it's how you shine, but among doctors it's how we tell others what is happening with our patients so that they continue to get good care when you are not in the hospital to provide it yourself. So let's go see our patients and tend to their needs and then I'm going to help you with the rest."

"Wait, I need to say something," Byron Weeks said as the subdued group started to rise from their chairs. "I may be out of line, and if so, then you can fire me. There's a job opening for a pastry chef down the street from my apartment that's looking pretty good to me now."

I smiled at his ability to create a glimmer of humor in what so far had been a joyless morning. It was unusual for an intern to speak up this early in the training year, but even the most docile of animals will strike back if poked enough with a stick.

"None of this is Dr. Singleton's fault and if he's not going to defend himself, I will. It's mad here. You can't get anything done. We admitted fourteen patients in the past day—eight of them after midnight. Four of my six new patients can't give me any history, so I desperately need their old charts. But the ward clerks tell us they are too busy to get them. Now that excuse might work during the day, but at two in the morning? We can't get admitting orders processed, nurses seem to disappear as soon as the sun goes down, and rumor has it that the sole respiratory therapist that works nights hasn't been seen for days. I had to scare up the parts to a nebulizer and figure out to make the thing work in order to give one of my patients a breathing treatment last night. It was either that or he would have gone without.

"Just to make sure that nobody had a good night, I admitted a problem patient. He's the guy with scleroderma. He's always in the hospital and has been driving his doctor crazy—he calls every day complaining of something. I don't think his doc knows what to do with him so he told him to come to the hospital. He was supposed to be here yesterday morning but didn't show up until a quarter to eleven last night. He was here five minutes before demanding that they open up the kitchen and fix him a meal because he had missed supper. Every fifteen to twenty minutes he was complaining about something. Nothing we gave him for pain worked. The nurses stopped answering his calls so the ward clerk called me. One of us was in that man's room all night. We couldn't take care of the other patients let alone work on our presentations."

Byron hung his head in frustration as his pager beeped for the third time in as many minutes. Both telephones in the conference room were ringing as the lights flashed on and off repeatedly. Looking up at the lights and shaking his head in bewilderment, he said, "How can you guys take this? It's just chaos here."

It felt good to get out of the conference room and to walk the medicine wards with my team. We would visit the bedside of each of our patients—sometimes to examine, sometimes to judge the effectiveness of treatment, and sometimes just to talk to the special people we would find there. While many of my colleagues would disagree, it was the best place for teaching. The bedside was where we practiced our science and if cure was to be found, it would be found there. Sometimes so much more was found there as well.

As our group stepped onto the main corridor of the medicine ward, the calm I had hoped to find there was nowhere in sight. Above almost every patient's room, a light flashed to indicate that the patient within needed assistance and had pressed the nurse call button. I wondered how long they had waited and how much longer they would have to wait. The hallway was narrow yet cluttered with dietary carts, empty gurneys, and abandoned wheelchairs. Another medical team struggled to pass an unhappy-appearing housekeeper that had chosen that time and that place to mop the floor. Spine-tingling alarms blared from monitors in the nursing station, but no one was there to notice.

"Yep," Byron Weeks mumbled, "it's just chaos here."

Peter Rockwell was a sixty-year-old man who spent many of his days homeless. He had family in town but he seldom saw any of them. Every couple of months when his COPD made it difficult to breathe, he would come to the VA. It was like a home to him. Even if he wasn't admitted, they always gave him something to eat.

The police had called the ambulance that brought Peter to the VA hospital. He had spent the night sleeping on a park bench and when they came to chase him away, discovered that he couldn't move. He could move his left arm some but everything else had been stilled. That arm trembled when we walked into his room. The air was heavy with fear—overwhelming fear.

I held the chest x-ray up to the light. His doctor was right. There was a huge mass in the right upper lobe of his lung and it was eroding several of his thoracic vertebrae, which had collapsed. The good news was that Mr. Rockwell was not in much pain. The rest of the news, however, was very bad. He most certainly had lung cancer, but that seemed to be the least of his problems. His spinal cord had been severely damaged and experience told us that such damage was usually permanent. He was placed on high doses of steroids to try to reduce spinal cord swelling and the neurosurgeons were on their way for urgent consultation. It was exactly as I would have done.

Nobody thought that Clark Kenston should have been admitted to the hospital. His son had brought the seventy-four-year-old man to the VA for an appointment with the dietician, but then refused to take him home afterwards. His father had been unusually tired recently and the family was worried that the colon cancer he had several years earlier was back. He wouldn't take no for an answer.

Mr. Kenston was already feeling better when we saw him on rounds. The only thing his doctors had done for him since being admitted to the hospital was to order that a catheter be placed into his bladder. The Kenston's didn't understand how that was going to make him feel less tired, but they were just glad that someone was taking their concerns seriously. His doctors expected the routine blood work that they had ordered to be normal and were surprised to find that Mr. Kenston was in renal failure. They were even more surprised when the catheter drained several liters of urine from his bladder, but they were also heartened—it was a cause of renal failure that they could treat.

"Good pick up, Dr. Singleton," I said as we were leaving Mr. Kenston's room. "Most doctors would have sent him home. Fatigue is an outpatient problem. What made you admit him?"

The young physician gave me a rueful smile. "Surrender," he said. "Simple surrender."

"I'm sorry," I said, not at all certain I had heard him correctly.

"You don't know how much I would like to tell you that there was an intelligent reason for admitting him, but there wasn't. We were so busy yesterday and didn't have time to admit him and I really didn't think there was anything wrong with him, but then again, I didn't have the time to fight with his son about it. I figured it was easier just to bring him in and send him home in the morning after we placated the family by running some tests.

"We still don't have labs back from this morning so it's anyone's guess if his renal function is better after placing the Foley catheter, but he certainly looks better. It gives me the chills to think I could have sent him home. His renal failure could have become permanent by the time anyone figured it out."

"Sometimes patients and family know best," I observed, "and it can drive docs nuts. But if you are willing to listen and are open to the possibility that we don't have all of the answers, a lot people can be helped. You may not find it in the textbook but there's a great deal of intelligence, and much wisdom too, in surrender. Not trying to control everything and everyone around us is hard for docs, but it is a powerful tool of healing."

You couldn't help but feel sad standing next to Sam Marshet's bed. The eighty-eight-year-old man had a litany of problems—COPD, hypertension, chronic renal failure, and heart disease—but it was heart failure that made life particularly difficult in recent years. His work of breathing had increased dramatically over the previous day and his family brought the stoic man—against his wishes—to the hospital. He would have preferred to remain at home and encounter what yet remained of his journey sitting in his worn recliner by the fireplace. The pump just couldn't circulate enough blood to his meet his body's needs. Hardly a body system was not affected. His lungs had filled with fluid, making breathing difficult. His kidneys barely functioned. When he was not sleeping, he wanted to.

Mr. Marshet's doctors were in a tough spot and perhaps for the very first time, had lived throughout a sleepless night the physicians' creed of *first do no harm*. Medicine to help clear the fluid from his lungs made the kidney failure worse. Medicine to help the kidneys caused the already low blood pressure to drop even lower. The potassium placed in the IV fluid—to replace that lost by the use of the diuretics—burned his veins and caused much pain. The oxygen mask was uncomfortable against his face.

His doctors could not cure and even their modest efforts at comfort seemed so little compared to the enormity of suffering that lay in that bed. Mr. Marshet's heart failure had reached its final stages, but his family was still not ready to let him go. Much life could have been lived along the journey that they were unable to travel with him. It was sad standing there by his bed.

He smiled at me for a long time before attempting to speak, his eyes moving from one tired-looking face to another among the team of doctors and students that circled his bed. His body was frail but there was strength in those eyes and wisdom that had been collected over a lifetime.

"You have quite a group of young doctors," he said softly. "You can be very proud of them. They were in here all night, you know. If one had to leave, someone else would take their place. They didn't have to do that—there wasn't anything that I needed—but to see such caring in other people made me forget I was sick. I realized how fortunate I am. I could have been like that poor guy down the hall. He screamed and carried on all night. The docs were constantly being called away for him, but by the sounds of it, I don't think they were able to do anything to help him. I'm glad I don't have what he has—to be so miserable. I hope you can help him."

He rested for a few breaths as he seemed to contemplate something of great importance. His gaze rested on his two daughters with tear-streaked faces that stood in the corner of the room. Turning back to me, he said, "Try to get me home. That's where I want to be. I think they finally want that too. Whether it's home or here, the important thing is that we are all together. We've always known that."

"But please," he said with surprising strength, "if you can't get me home, no machines."

I placed my hand on top of his and said softly, "We'll try to get you home, and no machines."

We stood outside Mr. Marshet's room for several minutes, each of us lost in private moments of thought. Words could not capture what happened in that room—and what obviously had taken place during the night—either in the written notes of admission documents or in a formal presentation on morning rounds. I looked at the incredibly young-looking faces that had gathered around me. Only their white coats betrayed the identify of doctor. Instead, I saw sons and daughters and granddaughters and grandsons each saddened by an old man that they could not cure. But while they did not yet understand, they had done so much more. Yes, I was indeed very proud of them.

Our thoughts were interrupted by a loud commotion at the end of the hall. The nursing supervisor tried desperately to silence one of her nurses before news of the ruckus spread throughout the hospital, but it was too late. A small crowd had already gathered, eager to learn more about the fight between the patient on 6-South and the VA nurse. Rumor had it that security had to be called.

"I don't care who he knows or who he'll call," the nurse loudly declared to all who would listen. "I don't have to take that from anybody. I don't care if he is a patient."

She was an older nurse and had been at the VA hospital as long as I could remember. Her training was old school and she was no nonsense about her work. She could recite every VA regulation from memory and compromise was not a word in her vocabulary. Patients—and more than a few doctors—were scared to death of her and it was hard to imagine anyone crossing her.

"Don't hush me," she snapped at the nursing supervisor. "That man threw a telephone at me. When that missed, he slapped me. There's no mistake. He was intent on assault. I want him arrested. They have medical facilities in prison."

"It's just chaos here," Byron mumbled as we approached the turmoil. "Don't tell me," he said to the nursing supervisor, "let me guess. Mr. Smitt?"

"Ronnie Smitt?" I asked in surprise.

"You know him?" Byron asked cautiously.

"No, but I heard the name," I said with a smile.

"Dr. Weeks," the nursing supervisor implored, "would you please explain to Nurse Parks that you haven't been able to get Mr. Smitt's pain under control and that we need to understand if he is irritable. You can't really blame the poor man."

"By any chance, did Mr. Smitt call your boss?" I asked the nursing supervisor.

"The nursing director," she replied with a touch of disbelief in her voice. "He's done it before. We need to keep this man happy. Heaven knows who he'll call next."

"He was going to call the chief of staff last night," Byron observed.

"He did," I said.

"How do you know that?" Byron asked.

"Because the chief of staff called me," I replied.

Byron's eyes grew wide and his face paled a bit at the thought. "I'm so sorry, sir," he said. "Had I known he was actually going to do it I would have figured out some way to make him happy."

Ronnie Smitt was indeed an unhappy man. It was obvious in everything about him when we entered his room—the grimace on his face, his folded arms and hunched-over posture, and even the way he mumbled to himself as he rocked forward and back on the edge of his bed. But there was more than unhappiness in that room. It was a sudden and overwhelming feeling, much like walking into the sweltering heat of summer from an air-conditioned room. I knew so very little about this man but already I felt an intense dislike toward him, and that bothered me.

With the team still streaming into his room and before I had a chance to introduce myself, he launched into an impressive array of complaints—his pain was being ignored, the food was not edible, the room was cold, the television did not work, he could not sleep, there was too much noise, the bathroom needed to be cleaned, the phlebotomist was incompetent, the nurses were rude, and his doctors were nothing more than children.

At thirty-eight, he was younger than I expected, and despite the hideous gown that made everyone look the same, there was a distinctiveness about him. He seemed to be a man that was used to being in control and accustomed to being listened to—something he was unlikely to find at the VA hospital.

"That's quite a list," I observed. "I have to give you a lot of credit. Most men would never be found in a place with all those problems. It takes a special man to be able to tough out such adversity. I could never do it."

Mr. Smitt sat there with a confused look on his face, his eyes blinking rapidly. For a brief moment, he was rendered speechless and I had the distinct impression that such things did not happen often to him.

"I know you don't feel good," I continued, "and I'm very sorry about that, but I have to tell you, Mr. Smitt, your strategy for getting better is not serving you. You may want to rethink the attack mode that you've been in. You see, when you play offense it makes others play defense. There are some wonderfully talented and dedicated people here. I've seen them create miracles. You need a miracle. It's hard to create one, or even be able to see one though, when you are always on the defensive.

"I just came from a wonderful man's bedside a couple of rooms down the hall. He wasn't able to sleep much last night because somebody was constantly complaining and raising a storm. This man is dying, but he wasn't thinking about himself this morning, he was thinking about you. He feels sorry for you and hopes that we can do something to help you.

"That's the kind of miracle that can be found here, but one that will never be able to penetrate the energy of anger that you have filled this room with. Nobody wants to come in here and I can't blame them. Healing is an energy too, but with all of the darkness you have wrapped yourself in, I'm not so sure you will ever feel it.

"We are going to do everything we can do to help you, sir, but if you are unhappy enough with your care that you find it necessary to disturb that old man down the hall again, then I'll sign the discharge papers myself and you can find a hospital that better meets your expectations."

Mr. Smitt never uttered a word while I was in his room but his eyes told me much. They were filled with anger. There was a story there that our history taking had missed, one that might make it possible to help this man but one that he was not yet ready to share. He had scleroderma, a disease I had not seen before in a man. Typical of the disease, it had struck during his prime working years and was marked with fibrosis and tightening of the skin, joint pain, and involvement of internal organs. His pain was much more severe than most and his many specialists were baffled as to why or how to adequately treat it.

"I would have sent him packing this very morning," his nurse snorted as we gathered outside Mr. Smitt's room to discuss his care.

"Look," I said, "he certainly has acted like a jerk, but in many ways we taught him how to be a jerk and encouraged him to be very good at it. When hospital administrators have a knee-jerk response to patients that complain, many patients are taught how to complain louder and more often. And while everyone scurries around to keep the complainer happy, we lose sight of what we are here for and you can't help people in that state. So our patients get even angrier and complain more. We have created that monster that sits in that bed, and as painful as it is for us, we need to try to help him.

"What we can't allow, though, is for him to interfere in the care of other patients, which is why I said what I did to him. I don't want to see him leave the hospital. He needs our help as much as Mr. Marshet. Unfortunately, I'm not sure just what that help might be."

The turmoil of the VA hospital churned on in the days to come but for the most part the young doctors on the team were simply too busy to notice. As hospital administrators and patient advocates struggled with the cosmetics of keeping Mr. Smitt happy, his doctors struggled with the substance of his disease. It was a disparity as stark as the construction work on the new hospital addition that I walked past every morning, but it was a symbolism that I would not appreciate at the moment.

Swimming in turbulent waters can be exhausting and working

at the VA was no less draining. By week's end, Peter Rockwell was in surgery to have his spine stabilized, the urologists had attended to Clark Kenston's urinary obstruction, and Sam Marshet had returned home to continue his journey. They were three lives that had been profoundly changed during the time they spent at the VA hospital, but the lives that they touched while there were changed as well.

The team seemed in unusually good spirits when I walked into the conference room early one morning, vigorously debating whether there might a pattern in the chaos of the VA. Mostly, they were just happy that Ronnie Smitt was going home. While he had stopped his complaining after my talk with him, he was returning home still an angry man and I feared that we had cured nothing. Clearly there had been little healing.

"So tell me about this pattern you see in chaos," I asked as I sat down at the conference room table with my cup of coffee.

"We were talking about the possibility that what appears to be chaos might not be just random events," said Bruce Singleton, "that there may be a pattern or even an intelligence involved."

"It's called the *Chaos Theory* and I'm not having any of it," scoffed Byron Weeks. "The only meaning in what happens in this place is that there is no meaning. You spend your day beating your head against the wall and the only thing that comes of it is a sore head. You can't corrupt science enough to put a good spin on the uncontrolled bedlam here."

"I thought the *Chaos Theory* was a spiritual principle?" asked one the medical students.

"Now that's helpful," Byron groaned sarcastically. "If science can't provide the answers, we're certainly not going to find them singing *Kumbaya*. Mr. Smitt came here with something medical science can't cure, but he keeps coming back again and again. If there were answers in spirituality, he wouldn't be leaving as the same mean and spiteful man in which he arrived, and as I am sure he will return for some other unfortunate medical team. Sometimes bad things happen—there's no other meaning than that."

"I don't know about that, Byron," I wondered aloud. "I used to think that science and spirituality couldn't be more diametrically opposite—that the presence of one made the other an impossibility—but the longer I practice medicine the more I find my science inadequate to explain what I encounter on a daily basis. Perhaps they are one in the same. Perhaps our science has only recently evolved enough to permit an understanding of spirituality. I'm struck by the realization that some of our greatest minds in science are deeply spiritual beings. What might they know that I should know, or that my patients would want me to know?

"It's hard to reconcile the design and precision that we find in the natural world with the randomness and coincidence that we perceive in our personal world. Perhaps we do not see the meaning, or the intelligence if you will, because we haven't been looking. We were never taught to look. Imagine what we might discover if we are open to the possibility that so much more exists than what we have been taught, what he have experienced, or even what we understand. I can't help but wonder if Mr. Smitt's disease is the scleroderma or the anger that he carries with him. As a doctor, I know how to approach the scleroderma but for the anger, I need more. Maybe that realization is the first step in helping Mr. Smitt and others like him."

It was rare to encounter discussion among doctors that touched upon the metaphysical and the epistemological—and that was a shame. Perhaps that was the meaning we struggled to find or refused to acknowledge in Ronnie Smitt's journey—that healing required a different way of looking at things.

Whether it was the contemplation that meaning might exist in chaos or simply the satisfaction of being rid of a difficult patient, it was good to see my team happy. I too was happy. It was my afternoon in the country.

Between teaching rounds every morning and maintaining a busy practice, months that I served as a medicine ward attending were extraordinarily hectic and many thought I should forgo the Friday afternoon clinic in the country. The free clinic in the hills of Appalachia was a two-hour drive from my office at the Teaching Hospital, but it was the antithesis of what medicine had become. Medications were limited, laboratory studies few, and diagnostic tests virtually nonexistent, but need was abundant as was the opportunity to listen and to touch. Despite the marvels of modern medicine and a practice in the midst of the best of the best, I often struggled at day's end to identify someone whom my efforts might have made a difference. That never happened in the clinic and strange as it seemed at the time, it was the patients that had come to see me there that made the difference—to me.

A most special part of the clinic was the medical residents that would join me there. It was a strange land for them—barren of technology and abundance that they had already grown accustomed to in medicine—and invariably they felt inept and uncomfortable. Without their tools of cure, they would discover healing—many for the first time.

The chaos of the VA hospital did not follow me to the clinic that day—angst and worry seldom did. Somewhere along the rise and falls of the twisting country roads, worry just melted away. I dreaded my commute to and from work each day and I almost always encountered what I focused my thoughts on: gridlock, ill tempers, and lost time. The greatest challenge in my trips to the country, however, was braking for turtles and more than once I stopped to move them from harm's way.

Often, a resident made the drive with me and I always delighted in their reaction to the incredible beauty that enveloped us along the way. It was so unlike what they experienced every day and the sudden reminder that a world existed outside of the hospital seemed to take them by surprise. I made the drive alone that day, the first-year resident having called to inform me that she had been delayed by a difficult patient in her own clinic. I was happy when she declined my offer to do the clinic without her—she sounded so harried on the telephone that I knew the afternoon in the country would do her good.

Together we saw hypertension, emphysema, coronary artery disease, and diabetes. They were maladies not unlike those encountered in the city—maladies that stubbornly resisted improvement despite the wealth of resources at our fingertips. In the scarcity of the country clinic, however, improvement was as improbable as it was dramatic. It was a paradox that was not lost even upon my young colleagues.

There was also depression in the clinic—depression masquerading as back pain, fatigue, and sadness. I watched with interest as a young mother left the clinic after an atypically long visit with the resident. She was smiling and had a look of hope about her, something I hadn't noticed on her arrival.

"It looks like that went well, doctor," I said to a preoccupied-looking Cathy Johnson.

"It did," she responded with a smile, obviously returning from another place in her thoughts. "She's been having headaches and almost constant fatigue for several months and was reluctant to consider depression a possibility. Here's this lady—her husband's dead, she's raising three kids alone, and is trying to live on $689 a month—and feels guilty about being depressed because there are so many people less fortunate than her. I didn't do anything but listen. She helped herself. Actually, she helped me as well."

She had been our last patient and I sat down with the young doctor in the now empty examination room. "Anything I can do to help?" I asked.

"No," she smiled again, "I was just thinking about another lady with depression that I saw this morning. In fact, she was the reason I was late. She didn't want to admit that she was depressed either, but she was. She had been having headaches as well and they got progressively worse until this morning when she couldn't take it any more. I found out that her husband was getting out of the hospital today."

"So her husband's been sick and she's been worrying about him," I surmised.

"No," Cathy said sadly, "she didn't want him to come home. She didn't want him to ever come home."

Maybe it was all of the teachers that had visited me along my journey, but I always knew when a special story was on the horizon and my curious look urged Cathy to continue.

"She's thirty-eight I believe," my young colleague continued, "and since her husband's been ill, she's been the breadwinner and supporting the family. It wasn't always that way. Her husband was so successful in business that she didn't need to work—so she stayed home to raise the kids. Getting back in the workforce has been a major stressor for her, particularly when she can't earn close to what they had grown accustomed to.

"He was the perfect husband. She wanted for nothing, but it wasn't the material things that made the difference. He would call her from work a couple of times each day. At least once a week he would return home at night with fresh flowers. They would spend hours talking—he did most of the listening. One weekend each month, the kids would stay with grandparents and he would take her to a special place. She never knew where they were going—one weekend it would be on a beach resort, the next might be skiing in Montana, or sometimes it was a hotel a mile or two from home—but it was always special.

"He was the perfect father. He attended every baseball and dance practice no matter how busy his schedule. He found time for camping trips and slumber parties. Their local PTA once even named him father of the year.

"All that changed when he got sick. He became bitter and complained about everything and anything. Nobody wanted to be around him any more. He didn't get along with people at work and when he started to lose the company customers, they fired him. He was constantly angry—at everyone, even the kids—and eventually drove away all of his friends and even his family. His own parents won't stop by to see the kids if he's around. They even suggested that she divorce their son—but what about their vows?

"She told me she cried hysterically when the doctor called from the hospital to tell her he was being discharged. It was so peaceful at home without him. She had hoped the peace would last longer for her children."

"How do you solve a problem like that?" Cathy asked. "We can give her medication for the headache, which I did, but antidepressants are not going to change her circumstances. There wasn't a thing

I could do for her. She left the office just as miserable as she was when she got there. Why does it seem so much easier out here? What is it about these patients?"

Her question took me by surprise—not its substance but in the awareness that the asking revealed. The parade of lives that cross physicians' paths is so swift and so lengthy that many barely notice. It is even more so for the young physician whose urgency to put their hard-earned secrets of cure into practice often blinds them to those whom they seek to cure. It is an awareness that can come only through seeing the person within the patient. It is a concept that I did not know how to teach. Perhaps it can only be discovered and it should not have come as a surprise to me that it would be found here.

"I'm not sure it is easier out here, Cathy," I said quietly, "in fact, I suspect most physicians—even the ones at the Teaching Hospital—would struggle mightily and bemoan how difficult it is to practice medicine here. Maybe it has nothing to do with the patients. Maybe it's you. I suspect you walked into every room this afternoon with expectations somewhat different than those at the Teaching Hospital. I'm willing to bet that you anticipated providing less and instead delivered much more. Here, it is more about healing. Certainly, you must have seen it in your last patient's face?

"I've learned so much about healing here—things that I've been able to take back to the city with me. This place has helped me become a better doctor. You say there was nothing you could do to help your patient this morning, but you are wrong. You took time to listen. That is a precious gift and a powerful tool for a physician, one that I suspect you are going to use much more of after your day here in the country."

Cathy smiled at the thought. The stress that I saw in her eyes earlier in the day was gone. I had been right. The day here had been good for her.

"Your patient from this morning," I asked, my curiosity getting the better of me, "what was her husband's illness?"

"Scleroderma," she replied. "I had never heard of a case in a man before, but I'm sure it happens."

"I'm sorry," I said, convinced that I had heard her wrong, "what does he have?"

"Scleroderma," she said again.

"What hospital?" I managed to ask through my startled disbelief.

"I believe she said it was the VA hospital," she said matter-of-factly. "Is there some meaning in that?"

Is there some meaning in that? It was a question I asked my equally stunned team the following morning on rounds.

"It's quite a coincidence," observed Byron Weeks, "but it's nothing more than that."

"But when is something just too incredible to be a mere coincidence?" asked Bruce Singleton. "What are the odds of our attending physician discovering such intimate and telling history about one of our most difficult patients in the middle of a free clinic in the country? What are the odds of two residents from the same training program—unbeknownst to the other—grappling with the effects of the same family tragedy, but from opposite perspectives? It's just mindboggling."

"Maybe doctors believe in coincidence," I suggested, "because it is less threatening than the alternative—that there is an order to the universe. I've believed in coincidence for most of my life, but I have to tell you, when you start to pay attention to the lives that cross your path in medicine, you come to realize that there are no coincidences.

We may not understand it, but there are no coincidences. There are no accidents."

"If everything is so ordered," argued a clearly frustrated Byron, "and there was some meaning in all of the chaos Mr. Smitt brought into our lives, why didn't this information about him come to us when we could have made some use of it?"

"I can't answer that, Byron," I responded. "Maybe being aware of the possibility that the inexplicable that surrounds us might simply be beyond our level of understanding—at least for the moment—is enough for us to know."

In the days that followed, the medical students and residents on my ward team lived the paradox that was the VA hospital, and I lived it with them. The frenzied construction that I walked past every morning seemed to underscore just how little things had changed through the years within the walls of the VA hospital. The tangled bureaucracy that stifled exceptional care exposed the heroic efforts of the countless souls that were determined to provide it. The busier the emergency room got and the longer the wait, the more appreciative the patients became. It was among the most difficult places I had ever worked and offered rewards that could be found in no other place.

Indeed, there was chaos. It came in the form of young men with the stress of the battlefield painfully fresh in their thoughts, of middle-aged men seeking a better reality through alcoholism and drug abuse, and of aging warriors with hearts laden by disease and memories of the past. Through the turmoil and burden of responsibility, I watched the young doctors on my team grow. I never found them ill prepared again, either in the quality of their work or the dance that tradition required them to perform.

Not many days after that afternoon in the country, morning

rounds were interrupted by a page from the emergency room.

"You're not going to believe this," Bruce Singleton said after hanging up the telephone in the nursing station on the medical floor, "but Ronnie Smitt's back. He's in the ER now. We're going to have to end rounds early."

"I knew this was going to happen," a disgusted-looking Byron Weeks said. "We're not going to go through this again, are we?"

Bruce and Byron had been in the emergency room for several minutes by the time I arrived. There was little I could offer that the emergency room physician couldn't, but I was interested in watching the interaction between Mr. Smitt and his frustrated doctors. The scene in the corner cubicle of the uncomfortably small emergency room took me by surprise.

The patient that I had never seen without a scowl on his face was not complaining this day. He looked bad. His skin was pale and clammy, his body shook uncontrollably, and he moaned incoherently. The cardiac monitor revealed an unusually fast heart rate while the automated blood pressure readings seemed impossibly low. A nurse worked on each outstretched arm desperately trying to start an intravenous line, the pile of discarded IV packaging cluttering Ronnie's bed testifying to one failed attempt after another. He would not survive without an IV.

A middle-aged woman—whom I assumed was his wife—stood at the foot of his bed and sobbed. She said that Ronnie had been sick for a couple of days but had refused to come to the hospital. It struck me as strange—he had always seemed to want to be in the hospital. So too did her tears—they were not for herself but for him.

I stood in the back of the room and watched my young colleagues work, feeling more than a little pride in them. Bruce effortlessly inserted a needle into Ronnie's neck and threaded a large intravenous catheter into a major vein deep within the chest through which life-sustaining fluids and medications would flow. Without the slightest hesitation, Byron guided a small catheter into an artery in his patient's wrist, enabling accurate blood pressure monitoring. Ronnie was examined head to toe, blood was drawn for laboratory tests, and a portable chest x-ray was obtained. Although Ronnie was unconscious, Byron spoke softly too him, explaining everything that was happening. There was compassion in his voice that I hadn't noticed before and it touched me deeply.

Ronnie was admitted to the intensive care unit with a diagnosis of sepsis—infection that overwhelms the body. As was often the case, the source of the infection was not known so his doctors made an educated guess when selecting what antibiotics would be administered intravenously. It's called empiric therapy—doctors just can't bear the thought of guessing.

Byron spent the night at Ronnie's bedside and most of the following day and the day after that. He was there when his patient developed respiratory distress and ordered the breathing treatments that brought him comfort. He was there when his patient's heart raced wildly out of control and ordered the medications that brought him calm. And he was there when his patient woke up, took his first sip of water, struggled with his first step to a chair, and when he first smiled.

It was late one evening when I stopped by to see Ronnie before heading home. He had been transferred to a regular hospital room several days earlier and would in fact be ready to return to his own home in a day or two. He was smiling when I entered his room.

"Mr. Smitt," I said with pretend surprise, "what's with the smile?"

His smile turned into a broad grin before his face turned serious.

"I owe you all an apology, but I'm afraid I've forgotten how to do it. It has been a long time."

"Can you stay a moment?" he asked while gesturing at a chair next to his bed. He seemed surprised when I sat down but also a little frightened as he appeared to struggle to find the words he was looking for. "I didn't think you would want to take care of me after last time."

"Is that why you waited so long to come back to the hospital?" I asked.

"Partly," he said softly. "I treated everyone here so badly. I couldn't stop thinking about that dying man you told me about, the one that was worrying about me when I was so busy worrying about myself. It's been a long time since others occupied my thoughts. It's been humbling and rather frightening to discover how others see me. The worst was going home and seeing my children. They were frightened of me. I don't think they wanted me there. I could feel my home slipping away from me and I didn't want to leave it again.

"The first thing I saw when I woke up in the intensive care unit was Dr. Weeks sleeping in a chair in the corner of my room. The nurse said he had been there all night. I hadn't cried in years—just too mean and angry I guess—but I did that day. My mother always used to talk about unconditional love but I never really understood what it was until that moment. It was sleeping in my chair."

Some movement caught my eye and I looked up to see Byron Weeks standing in the doorway. He looked uncomfortable and tried to slip out unnoticed. "Dr. Weeks," I said in a loud voice, "shouldn't you be home?"

Before Byron had a chance to respond, his patient quickly said, "Didn't you know? He comes in every night. He spent a couple of hours playing cards with my wife and I last night. Not once did he mention my illness and it wasn't until he left that my wife and I realized we hadn't either. In those hours, it didn't exist. That gave us a lot to talk about. Why couldn't what happened last night happen today or even tomorrow? This morning everything seemed so clear—the way things used to appear to me. I realized how much I want to go home, how much I have waiting for me there, and how much my family wants me there.

"When I came to the hospital, I was so certain there was a medication or a treatment that would help me and I was so angry that you wouldn't give it to me. Help came from none of those things. I once said that my doctors were not much more than children. Where do children find such wisdom?"

It was one of those magical moments in medicine—moments that probably happen with regularity if only we are aware enough to notice—and I was determined that it wouldn't slip by uncelebrated. Byron would have much preferred that we walk in silence when we left Ronnie's room that night, but I just couldn't resist probing the freshly turned soil to see what might be growing there. "You do good work, Dr. Weeks," I said.

"I didn't do that!" exclaimed Byron, coming to a sudden stop just in front of the darkened nursing station.

"Sure you did," I said softly. "That's a different man in that room than we saw earlier this month. Is that just a *coincidence*? And the way you look at him seems a little different as well. Why the change?"

He smiled when I said *coincidence*, but his eyes quickly turned sad. "I haven't felt very good about myself the past few days. Maybe I'm just trying to exorcise my guilt for the way I thought about him. He was so sick in the emergency room and in desperate need of help, but he needed help before and I couldn't see it and so I didn't give it to him—not that I would have known what to do to help him. Imagine your children not wanting you to come home.

"All I did was spend time with him—it's not like I prescribed anything—and I think I did that more for myself than for him."

"Prescriptions can cure, Byron," I said. "It's among the many things in medicine that we learn while training to become a doctor. What you gave Mr. Smitt was much more powerful. You gave him time—a part of yourself—and through that gift Mr. Smitt found healing. You didn't learn to do that in medical school. Was it coincidence that you just happened to offer what he needed the most or was it something more?

"Mr. Smitt still has scleroderma but I don't think he will ever look at his disease the same way again. I have a feeling that going forward he's not going to allow his diagnosis to interfere with life anything like it has in the past. I don't know any other way to describe this than healing.

"Byron, just because you benefited from your interaction with Mr. Smitt doesn't make what you did less valuable. We help ourselves by helping others. While I suspect that helping Mr. Smitt has made you feel good—as well it should—I believe the greatest profit lies in the lessons he helped you learn, even if you don't understand them now."

I had no illusions that the lessons of Ronnie Smitt would linger long in the thoughts of his young doctor, for thoughts are fleeting and fragile things in medicine that dissolve rapidly in the pool of need and urgency in which we are constantly immersed. But there could be no mistake that those lessons touched his life and were most certainly left behind as seeds that one day would sprout and bear special fruit. Until then, it would be enough to know that he would never look at chaos quite the same way—to be open to the possibility that there was more. In that awareness, he would discover healing.

As I sat lost in the flight of the spicebush swallowtail, my thoughts turned to the journey that I had long ago shared with Bruce Singleton and Byron Weeks. I pondered what kind of physicians they had become and whether their special teachers had yet come alive and filled them with the wonder of a healing life as happened for me in this place. The butterfly's flight was indeed chaotic—filled with purpose and great beauty.

CHAPTER 7

Dying Saved my Life

To see the world in a grain of sand, and to see heaven in a wild flower,
hold infinity in the palm of your hands, and eternity in an hour.

WILLIAM BLAKE

It's only when we truly know and understand that we
have a limited time on earth—and that we have no way of
knowing when our time is up—we will then begin to live
each day to the fullest, as if it was the only one we had.

ELISABETH KUBLER-ROSS

I had never started an IV on a child before and my hand trembled as the needle slipped beneath the skin of the boy's left arm before entering the vein that had looked so much larger just moments before. It hadn't been a particularly bad fall and I was somewhat surprised that the school had called for the ambulance, but ours was a conservative community that took no chances when it came to their children. The coach that hovered anxiously over us seemed surprised that we were going to take the young football player to the hospital and downright dismayed that we would administer treatment before his parents arrived.

My partner and I had been paramedics for only a few months and there was very little we were certain of—that the smiling fourteen-year-old was fit to return to practice was not among them. He was tackled after receiving a pass and landed on the ball when he fell. We never learned in school about the diagnosis that the coach was certain of—getting the wind knocked out of you—and were even less thrilled with *walking it off* as an acceptable treatment. Aside from the purple bruise on the left side of his upper abdomen and his quickening heart rate, it was impossible to find much wrong with the young man, yet we insisted that he go to the hospital.

Even our driver—an unflappable twenty-year veteran of the fire service—silently questioned the wisdom of our actions. What he thought would be a leisurely drive to the hospital, however, became much more. We had barely driven a mile when our patient suddenly lapsed into unconsciousness. His pulse became weak and rapid, his blood pressure dropped precipitously and his abdomen became distended and rigid. A team of doctors and nurses were waiting for us when the ambulance pulled up to the emergency room. Within a half-hour, our patient was in surgery for a ruptured spleen. He did not play football that year, but he did the following year.

The emergency room was a mysterious and intimidating place for medical students and I felt as awkward and inept as any of my colleagues during my first clinical rotation there. I was amazed daily by the number of people that sought care for chest pain. While most would be found to have something other than heart disease as a cause of their distress—chest wall muscle strain, gastroesophageal reflux, pleurisy, or even anxiety—enough of them did that I had to fight the urge to rush out and have my cholesterol checked.

It was my fifth chest pain patient that day and it was barely noon.

My task was to obtain their medical history and perform their initial physical examination. Gwen Hawkman's story was no different than the four patients that had preceded her, yet the triage nurse had immediately placed her in one of the critical care rooms rather than a regular ER bed that the others had been assigned. Her examination was no different than the others either, except that she was a good two decades younger than my other patients had been.

I was just about to ask her nurse why the special treatment when Gwen developed the most curious look on her face, fell silent, and appeared to stare off into space. The squealing monitor above her bed revealed ventricular tachycardia—my years as a paramedic had taught me that much—and the emergency sprang into action. While there was urgency in the well-practiced routine, there wasn't panic. There didn't even seem to be much surprise. Gwen was fortunate to be in the right place at the right time, although even then I was able to recognize that her fortune had help. By evening, she had had emergency bypass surgery.

My last patient of the morning was just leaving the examination room when Erin, my nurse, shyly walked up to me with a sheepish grin on her face. The morning schedule had run late and I was anxious to get some lunch before the afternoon's patients started to arrive. Erin told me that Mabel Cramfield was waiting to be seen. She was among our legion of the worried well and always had a concern about her health. She walked into the office unexpectedly worried about a headache that woke her from her sleep that day. The elderly widow was such a pleasant person that Erin just couldn't turn her away.

Headaches were a common problem in our practice and Erin was hopeful that it wouldn't take much time to reassure Mrs. Cramfield and to send her on her way. But nothing happened quickly with

Mabel and Erin knew that lunch was doomed. She was still on the telephone with the deli down the street ordering take-out when I rushed out of the exam room. She looked at me in disbelief when I asked her to schedule an urgent MRI of the head. I couldn't have been with Mabel more than a minute or two—certainly not long enough to determine that such a test was warranted—but Erin never questioned such things and promptly set about making my wishes happen. By the time we finished seeing patients that evening, Mabel was being prepped for neurosurgery to repair the aneurysm that the MRI had detected in her brain.

It was my most valuable clinical skill and the hardest to learn. It was impossible to teach. Somewhere in their shaping, nurses, doctors, and even paramedics learn to distinguish between those who are sick and those who are not or whose needs are less urgent. We call it the clinical impression. It was the measure by which young doctors were evaluated at the Teaching Hospital. It made curing possible—sometimes it even made it look easy.

The teachers along my journey have helped me recognize a different kind of awareness—one that reaches deep into the essence of the lives that crosses our paths. Be it intuition, an inkling, or just a funny feeling, there can be no mistake that it is a spiritual impression, one with the power to guide and to transform. If the clinical impression is my most valuable clinical skill, this spiritual impression has become my most valuable healing skill. It cannot be taught, nor can it be learned. It can only be experienced. Jerry Ruchmund helped me experience it.

I hadn't seen Jerry Ruchmund in the office for almost two years. The forty-one-year-old construction worker didn't have health insurance and it limited his visits to only those of the greatest necessity.

He once joked that he would only be seen in a doctor's office if he was dying. Rachel made the appointment and insisted that he see his doctor. Had she not ridden in the car with him and accompanied him into the exam room, he probably wouldn't have kept his appointment.

Jerry and Rachel's relationship was a special one. While not husband and wife, they were much more than girlfriend and boyfriend. They had each struggled with a life of scarcity and unhappiness before meeting, and while life still seemed cruel at times after they had moved in together, it was so much better than facing the world alone. They developed a closeness seldom achieved though marriage. Their troubled lives had found peace together.

A cold chill swept through me when I walked into the examination room and saw Jerry sitting with Rachel. My skin tingled with goose bumps and there was a heaviness in the pit of my stomach. I knew the instant I saw him. I could see it in his eyes. I could feel it in the grasp of his hand. I could hear it in his voice. I didn't understand how, but I knew—every fiber of my being knew—that I was looking at a dying man.

Jerry had been having trouble with indigestion. He thought the problem had only been around for several months, but Rachel insisted that he had been complaining about it for well over a year. They both agreed it had grown worse over the past few weeks. Antacids used to help, but now the relief they brought only lasted for a few minutes. The burning was worse at night when he would lie down to sleep, so much so that he had been sleeping in a recliner in the living room for the past week. Although Jerry denied it, Rachel was certain he was having trouble swallowing.

Jerry's examination was unimpressive. He had lost twenty pounds since his last visit but considering the healthy diet Rachel had imposed on his life and the long walks they had been taking at night, it did not concern me. Perhaps his upper abdomen was slightly tender when I examined him. My clinical impression was of gastroesophageal reflux. His symptoms were classic and it was a diagnosis that a junior medical student would have been expected to make. It was also easy to treat. Normally, I would have stopped after prescribing a medication to block acid production in the stomach. Only if the symptoms had not improved after several weeks would I have investigated further, but that other impression troubled me. While I didn't understand it, I couldn't dismiss it.

While Jerry and Rachel waited for me in the examination room, I called a gastroenterologist that had done his internship with me at the Teaching Hospital. I had referred many patients to him over the years and he didn't hesitate a moment before agreeing to the favor I asked of him—even though he wasn't sure it was necessary. He would perform an upper endoscopy on Jerry to examine his esophagus and stomach and he would do it the following morning.

Jerry and Rachel both looked relieved when I reviewed the plan with them. Rachel was happy I was taking care of Jerry and Jerry was happy I was making Rachel happy. I was grateful that they did not appreciate how unusual it was to have endoscopy scheduled so quickly and they left the office optimistic that the medication I prescribed would help.

I was still doing morning rounds when I received a page from the endoscopy suite of a local hospital. I had expected my colleague to call after Jerry's procedure, but the earliness of the hour took me by surprise.

"I just finished scoping Mr. Ruchmund," he told me. "How did you know?"

"How did I know what?" I asked in a confused voice.

"With his symptoms," he went on, "I never would have scoped him. I would have treated him first."

"How did I know what?" I asked again, growing alarmed by the tone of my friend's voice.

"That he has esophageal cancer," he said. "It will take a couple of days to get the biopsy results back, but I don't need the biopsy to tell me that it's cancer. The tumor is huge. It involves over half of the esophagus. It's been in there working away for some time. I can't imagine that it is operable.

"I'm going to get a CT scan today and send him back to you in two days. Hopefully, the biopsy results will be back by then. You can decide the next step. If the scan looks okay, he'll need a surgeon, but if it looks as bad as I think it will then maybe an oncologist can help. His esophagus is so narrowed already that I doubt he will be able to eat much longer. I can put a feeding tube in when the time comes."

"Does he know?" I asked.

"No, he's still sleeping," he said. "With the anesthesia he's not going to remember anything that I tell him. I'm just going to tell him and his girlfriend that I found a growth in his esophagus and that you would know more after the biopsy results came back."

I can't say I was surprised when I hung up the phone. I didn't know that the answer would be esophageal cancer, only that the news was going to bad. I didn't relish the conversation that I was going to have to have in a couple of days, but was grateful that Jerry and Rachel would hear it from me rather than a stranger. It was a small thing, but when you had so little to offer it was the small things that seemed to matter the most.

Indeed, the news was bad. The biopsy confirmed the tumor was cancer. The CT scans that I held up to the light clearly showed the spread of tumor to nearby organs that the radiologist noted in his report. He also had tumors in his liver—most likely spread from the esophagus. I set the scans down on the desk in the examination room and sighed deeply as I peered into the eyes of Jerry and Rachel who sat breathlessly across from me.

After many moments of silence, Jerry swallowed and said, "It's okay, doc, we know it's cancer. We knew when the specialist said he found a growth. We've been reading everything we can find about it on the computer. We don't understand much of it but it sounds like it can be cured if they cut it out. Am I going to be able to have surgery?"

"I don't think so, Jerry," I said softly. "It's already spread too far. But we are going to send you to an oncologist to see if chemotherapy or radiation will help."

"And that will cure him?" Rachel asked anxiously.

"No," I said, "but it can slow the progression and reduce some of the impact on everyday life."

Jerry sat back in his chair, took a deep breath, and let it out slowly. "How long do I have, doc?" he asked. "Some of those sites we looked at made it sound like I only have a year. I have to have more time than that, don't I?"

"I never know how to answer that question, Jerry," I said. "The oncologist will discuss treatment options with you and many of them have been shown to prolong life. Some have more side effects than others, and you will have to weigh the extra time that they might give you against how they will make your feel. Longer life is not always a comfortable life. Only you will know what is best, but we will help you make a decision.

"The articles you read and the numbers that the oncologist will give you are just statistics. They only provide a picture of what the typical patient has experienced in the past. They are not predictions of the future. I don't have the wisdom to tell you how long you are going to live, only that your life is going to be far too brief. But you know, Jerry, life is short for everyone. There is no guarantee of tomorrow. Having cancer doesn't protect you from being killed in an automobile accident today. Maybe it's more important to get the most of every day rather than spend it thinking about how long tomorrow might last.

"If there are things that you and Rachel have wanted to do—do them now. If there is family that you haven't seen—see them now. If there is a friend that you have wanted to say something special to—say it now. If there is a place where you have found peace—go there now, because life is short."

Life would indeed be short for Jerry and the road would be bumpy. He and Rachel liked the oncologist that I sent him to. They found him easy to talk to and very honest in what the future most likely had in store for the two of them. They decided on a chemotherapy regimen that seemed to fit the couple best—mild in side effects even if the likely benefits would only be modest.

Every week or so Rachel would call me at home to update me on Jerry's progress. She had an incredible knack of calling at the most inopportune time—in the middle of a rare nap, sitting down to the first hot meal in days, while in the shower, or while savoring silence. I was chagrinned when I found her calls annoying as I recognized early on that her calls were not for Jerry but for herself. Rachel was one of my many teachers—it took so little time to bring a moment of comfort to another.

I still had toothpaste in my mouth as I rushed to grab the ringing telephone before the caller was directed to my answering machine. It was late—well past my typical bedtime—and any call at such an hour would certainly be urgent. I groaned when I recognized Rachel's voice on the other end of the line. She seemed oblivious to the lateness of the hour—an awareness that irritated me. Her speech was rushed and pressured as she tried to relate more information than I was capable of receiving—even wide awake.

"Rachel," I said in a sharp voice, "you need to start over and slow down. I can't understand you."

"It's Jerry," she said, sobbing, "he's a nervous wreck. You have to give him something that will calm him down so that he can rest."

Anxiety was not a stranger to my practice. It visited often and in many forms, but I had difficulty picturing it in Jerry. "That doesn't sound like him, Rachel," I said. "Tell me why you think it's his nerves?"

"He just can't sit still. He fidgets so much that it makes me nervous watching him. He feels like a blanket is smothering him and much of the time he acts like he can't catch his breath."

"How long has this been going on?" I asked with building apprehension.

"He woke up this way at six this morning," she said. "He was fine last night."

"Rachel," I asked in disbelief, "he's been like this all day and you wait until midnight to call me?"

"I'm sorry," she said, "I know it's late. I was going to call several times earlier today but he just threw a fit when I tried. I just couldn't take it any more. I just had to call."

"It's alright, Rachel," I said in the most comforting voice I could muster, "I wasn't in bed yet. I just don't like the idea that he might have needed help for the past eighteen hours and wouldn't accept it. If you couldn't call for him you would have been welcome to call for yourself. It sounds like you could have used some help yourself. Tell me about his shortness of breath."

"He's pretty comfortable when he's sitting quiet, but he just can't sit long before he wants to get up and pace the floor. It doesn't take many steps for him to be panting like a dog. It's worse when he lies down and tries to rest. He sits bolt-upright gasping for air with the most terrified look on his face. Can you give him something to calm him down?"

"I don't think this is anxiety, Rachel," I told her. "Jerry needs to be in the hospital. I don't want you to try to drive him so go ahead and call the ambulance."

I had yet to find restful sleep that night when the telephone rang again, this time from the emergency room attending physician. I was not surprised when she told me that Jerry's oxygen saturation in his bloodstream was very low and that his symptoms improved dramatically when he was placed on oxygen. A CT scan revealed a large blood clot had traveled to his lungs and was obstructing blood flow. It was called a pulmonary embolism and it was not uncommon in cancer patients. It was amazing that he had survived the day.

Jerry was admitted to the Teaching Hospital and placed on blood thinners. He would not stay in the hospital long, being able to walk the halls comfortably without oxygen after just two days. He found great humor in the fact that he was being sent home with blood thinning medication that was the active ingredient in rat poison. He thought it added a little extra color to his life.

While I hadn't thought it possible, Rachel kept even closer track of Jerry after that. With the increased scrutiny, the telephone calls became more frequent and either I had surrendered to their importance or they started to come at more thoughtful times, but they would never again be an annoyance. It was one such telephone call when she told me how unusually tired Jerry had been feeling and how black his stools had become. It was an ominous observation in a patient on blood thinners and it earned Jerry another trip to the hospital, this time for a bleeding duodenal ulcer.

The blood transfusions made Jerry feel like a new man and he returned home with energy that he had almost forgotten was possible. He and Rachel walked for hours in the nearby woods. It was spring and it had been years since they enjoyed the wildflowers that filled them with happiness but somehow stopped having time for.

It was bright yellow eyes that peered at Rachel one morning that prompted yet another stay at the Teaching Hospital. Tumor had spread to the liver and pancreas and blocked bile from reaching the intestines. After that, it was a bout of pneumonia. Despite a diagnosis that changed his life, the hospitalizations, and the obvious pain, I never heard Jerry complain. He always seemed more concerned about the impact his disease was having on Rachel than on himself.

The sun had yet to rise one Sunday morning and I lay in bed frustrated. I couldn't sleep. Days off were rare things in medicine and those free of deferred commitments and family obligations were exceptional. The day had been long planned in my thoughts. It would be spent reading, listening to music, and birding—but it would start by sleeping late. Typically, my day would start with the urgent prodding from the alarm clock, but on this morning, I was wide awake a good hour before the time I routinely, and often reluctantly, rose. Wishing sleep to return did little good and with a bit of a grumble, I decided to start my day early.

The eastern sky was just starting to lighten when I could feel my back porch beckon. It had been a long time since I had sat there and I wasn't quite sure why. With a steaming cup of coffee, I sat and watched the birth of a new day, lost within the golden hues of light and the wakening chorus of spring songbirds. I had no idea how long I had sat there—the sun was already peering over the tops of distant trees—when I heard the telephone ring. I could only smile when I saw the caller's number displayed on the telephone's screen. But it wasn't Rachel's voice that I heard when I answered.

"Jerry," I said in surprise, "is everything okay?" It was the first time he had ever telephoned me.

"Everything's great, doc," he said. "I hope I'm not calling too early, but I had a feeling you were up."

"Actually, I've been up a couple of hours," I observed, "but the strange thing is that I had wanted to sleep in today. Maybe I was just waiting for your call. What can I do for you, Jerry?"

"I just called to say thanks," he said softly. "It's hard to talk when Rachel is around, so while she's out in the kitchen making butterscotch pudding, I thought that I would give you a call. She has your number on our speed dial."

"Butterscotch pudding?" I asked

"Yep, she had people driving all over town yesterday looking for it," he laughed. "It's been hard for me to eat so she has tried every soft food she can think of. The thing is, I used to love butterscotch pudding as a kid. I forgot all about it. I sort of wish she would have thought about it a little earlier.

"It's time for me to go, doc. I'm not going to get that year, but you knew that the first day we sat in your office. I could see it in your eyes. Having that year was so important to us, but you helped us see that fully living a single day was more important. Rachel and I have talked for hours—often all night long. We've listened to music and read to each other. We've sat outside and watched the stars for hours—until those stars spoke to us. We've lived more in five weeks than I would have lived in a lifetime. I thought I knew what love was, but it's more than anything I had ever experienced or could have ever thought possible. I would have spent my life without knowing what life was all about.

"Dying saved my life, doc. I wanted you to know and I wanted to say thanks."

I'm not sure how long I sat there holding the silent telephone to my ear before I realized that Jerry had gone. I had become lost in the magnificence of his words, no less stirring than the splendor I had watched unfold around me that morning. I was taken back to an earlier time when a young doctor made butterscotch pudding for her patient and marveled in the coincidence that I knew was so much more. I had planned to have a special day, and it was.

I was lost in the world of cure when Rachel's visit the following morning reminded me that it was but a small part of a healing life. She smiled at the crowded waiting room and promised that she would not keep me long. She didn't want me to hear of Jerry's passing that weekend over the telephone.

"I'm doing fine," she said when I asked how she was handling his loss, "and I'm rather surprised by it. But I was ready for it and so was he. Once we got past the shock and sort of surrendered to what was—something he worked hard to get me to see—we didn't have to worry about the future and what was left was more wonderful than anything I could have imagined. I fell in love with a man that I thought I had already loved."

"You know he called me yesterday?" I asked her.

"Oh, that's not possible," she said. "The past few days he was too weak to get out of bed let alone use the phone."

"Sure it is. He told me you were making butterscotch pudding," I insisted.

Rachel's eyes grew wide and she covered her mouth with her hand. Her hand trembled softly. "I was making pudding yesterday morning," she observed with a whisper, "but I didn't think he knew. I wanted to find something that would make him happy, but I was too late. But how could he have called you?"

"You weren't too late, Rachel," I said. "He found happiness and he found it with you. I don't know how he called me. Perhaps I was dreaming, but then how would I have known about the pudding? There is much that I come upon that I can't explain. The minute the logical part of me stops trying to understand everything that I encounter the more I encounter that which I do not understand. Not understanding it doesn't make it less real, but it does make it special. I watched the sunrise yesterday. Its beauty left me spellbound yet I do not understand what makes all of the colors or causes the birds to sing even before it starts to get light."

Rachel smiled because she didn't understand all that had happened in the weeks that had passed, but they had been very special and would change the way she looked at life forevermore. Jerry's dying had saved her life.

CHAPTER 8

Do I Know You?

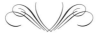

The one exclusive sign of thorough knowledge is the power of teaching.

ARISTOTLE

Millions of Spiritual Creatures walk the earth unseen,
both when we sleep and when we awaken.

JOHN MILTON

The action that swirled around me in the nursing station fascinated me. It was change day—no different than the scores of other change days I had witnessed at the Teaching Hospital but paid little notice of. Perhaps it was the passage of time or maybe the influence of special teachers that had shared part of their journey with me, but those things I knew the best and understood the most somehow seemed different. There was a depth to the flow of life—both that of patient and of caregiver—that I hadn't noticed before. Much of our medicine was practiced in the shallows of those waters—it was where cure was found—but it would be in the stillness of its depths where the discovery of healing was possible.

There was chaos to be sure—harried nurses, stressed ward clerks, and struggling doctors-in-training—but there was a hidden order that I hadn't appreciated before and my thoughts turned to those early days at the VA hospital when chaos made learning possible. In the apparent randomness of nursing reports, debates over patient management, and teaching, there was a beauty like that of an unrehearsed symphony. It was the teaching—the ancient ritual passed down from the days of Hippocrates—that touched me particularly strong this day.

While the principles of medicine are gleaned from texts and honed in lecture halls, much of the science of medicine is learned from those that come before us. With the lessons comes a connection to the past and the perpetuation of tradition. We are taught to honor old and cherished ways and to think as we have always thought. As I looked around the nursing station that day, I marveled as tradition unfolded just below the din of the chaos.

Teachers were everywhere. A seasoned colleague stood near the fax machine discussing with a senior resident the essential components of a preoperative consultation in an elderly patient. A frustrated-looking junior resident listened intently as his team leader explained the calculation of serum osmolality in a dehydrated patient for what must have been the third time. At the corner table, a junior resident patiently helped an intern determine the proper dosage of antibiotics in a lady with renal failure. Everyone teaches everyone else in medicine. It's how we learn to cure disease.

I couldn't hide my delight at seeing Sam again. Obviously, starting a rotation on one of the ward teams, I was thrilled with the prospect of seeing more of this young doctor who had touched my heart and reminded me of the importance of dreams. She sat at an adjoining table with a third-year medical student—the look of fright in his eyes was unmistakable—and he hung on every word she said with eagerness and a bit of awe. She was his teacher and the realization brought a smile to my face.

Students come and well-trained physicians leave with such frequency at the Teaching Hospital that it is easy not to notice the miraculous transformation that is the essence of our work there. With rituals rooted in ancient times and technology newly discovered, students become physicians with breathtaking speed. I could see it so clearly in Sam. She had grown so much in so little time. Now she had become a teacher and I longed to know what lessons she might have to offer her young charge.

They were discussing a patient they were preparing to discharge from the hospital on medication for high cholesterol. Sam taught not from textbooks—she had grown past such things—but from empathy and practicality. It was something that many attendings were unable to do.

"I just don't understand why we need to know about Mrs. Clayton's finances?" her student said. "Shouldn't we be blind to such things? Everyone should receive the best we have to offer, whether they are an industry CEO or are homeless. Let's just send her out with that new statin. It's supposed to be the best. Asking about her income is just going to embarrass her and make her feel poor."

"I used to think, until quite recently in fact," Sam said with a faraway look in her eyes, "that to be professional was not to pry into the personal lives of our patients and not to ask questions that might embarrass them. But now I wonder whether such advice is simply expedience—to protect us from venturing into areas that we simply do not have time for. Practicing evidence-based medicine is all the rage now. Maybe we need to practice practical-based medicine as well. Sometimes I wonder whether the number crunchers that produce all of the guidelines have ever sat with a patient and looked them in the eye.

"Not long ago I saw a man in a clinic. It was a free clinic out in the country. Mr. Weaver was his name. He passed out one day and was taken to the emergency room. The doctor found a bruit in his neck, but Mr. Weaver couldn't afford to have a Doppler ultrasound done on his carotids, so the doc put him on something to thin his blood. Mr. Weaver's social security—his only income—was $623 a month. The prescription would have cost him over $150 a month. I asked Mr. Weaver why he accepted a script for a medicine that he knew he couldn't afford to fill and he told me he didn't want to embarrass the doctor. The doctor wanted to help him and he didn't want to deprive him the opportunity to give.

"I learned so much that day; things that I don't know how you can be a doctor without knowing about. None of it we read about in school or hear about in conferences. I guess the important lessons never are. Mr. Weaver is going to be with me every time I see a patient. When I write a prescription, I see his face and wonder how I can do better."

There may not have been much science in what Sam taught but there was great wisdom. If the science of medicine was taught by our predecessors, then the art of medicine was something to be discovered along our journey. Some physicians discovered it early while others never would grow beyond journal articles and grand rounds. A few of the special ones would share the excitement with others—like Sam had done with her student—so that they too might look for, and be enriched by, the wisdom that could be found in their patients.

The sadness I had once seen in Sam was gone and despite the bedlam that defined change days at the Teaching Hospital, there was an unmistakable calm about her. Indeed, she looked happy and it stood in stark contrast with the energy that surrounded her. As I looked about the room, I realized that she had been right that day in the clinic—nobody looked happy. The students, well they always looked a bit terrified. Fatigue seemed to plague the faces of the residents, although more than a little loneliness could be seen as well. The sober-faced attendings were mired in the routines of their day—unaware that they were teaching.

It was an unusual place to find beauty—in the midst of chaos—but it was there. Carved from the consciousness focused on cure and treatment was a tiny sliver of something different; that perhaps we could be more than we had been taught. It wasn't a new idea—its wisdom was as timeless as the universe—but its presence in the Teaching Hospital was as unexpected as it was hopeful. Our greatest teachers are our patients and we can share their lessons—how to heal—with others.

There was something almost spiritual in the way Sam spoke to her student and the warmth I felt was no different than that which nourished me in the magical light of Demazie Hollow. Spirituality isn't something that I expected to find when I embarked upon a career of caring for patients, and medical education did nothing to prepare me for the possibility that healing required more than that which could be prescribed or be performed by a physician's hand. Even in my early days as a paramedic though, there always seemed to be something more in my patients' touch or in their stories—more than the textbooks wrote about, more than lecturers spoke about, and more than my mentors told me would be possible. But my teachers have been patient and have made the journey with me. One of those teachers was Jacob Keller.

Jacob Keller was fifty-six years old when he first came to my office. His wife, Janice, was sitting with him when I walked in the examination room. They had been married some thirty-five years and I had the feeling there was never a time when she hadn't been at his side. I had seen it before and it was always special. It was not the first time I would look at two individuals and see only one. Theirs was a permanent bond, forged through every rise, and especially every fall, of the journey they had walked together. What once made them distinct—personality, tastes, and even political persuasion—had been burned away in the crucible of life experience to reveal the pureness of a single soul. It would be many years before I would recognize just how similar were the souls of my many special teachers that had touched my life—as if they shined from a single light.

Jacob was a self-employed tradesman. Working from a shop in his home, he built a successful living out of doing what he loved to do. A cabinetmaker by trade, he hand made furniture for his customers' homes. He was not the fastest worker, but there was none better. He did one piece of furniture at a time and refused to move on to the next job until everything was perfect. He considered it sacred work. He felt a special energy with every project and felt humbled by the opportunity to add a part of himself to each piece of furniture that he made.

He was a quiet and stoic man. Janice always did the talking for both of them. It was just the way it had always been, just as it was for other things. She did the shopping; he kept the finances. She charmed the customers on the phone and in the office; he stayed in the shop. He cooked while she cleaned. One was not complete without the other.

It took many visits for Jacob to grow comfortable enough to allow me an occasional peak under the shell that he had spent a lifetime building. Much of what I learned about him I learned through Janice. Each office visit revealed another shard of information about the man, much like a jagged-shaped piece of a jigsaw puzzle. As the pieces of the puzzle slowly came together, the picture of a kind and generous man emerged. There was a shyness about him, one that made it difficult for him to share much with others. He relied on his hands and the creations they created in his shop to speak for his heart, and judging from what his customers told me about his work, his heart was immense and filled with great beauty.

As months dissolved into years, Jacob and Janice's office visits gradually required more and more time to complete. We would find ourselves lost in conversation about family, travel, and the many small things that tend to make life uniquely special. Somewhere along the way, we discovered we had become friends. Their presence on my office schedule always made for a good day and on each visit, I looked forward to learning something new about Jacob—and I always did. Still, I couldn't help but feel that there was so much more to learn.

Jacob and Janice were seldom ill and their visits to the office were typically spent managing modest elevations in blood pressure and blood cholesterol levels. It seemed only natural that they would both have the same health problems and take the same medications. It always seemed that hypertension and hypercholesterolemia were concessions that Jacob reluctantly made to Janice and that he would go no further. He simply refused to consider illness a possibility. Aches were the product of a hard day's work and pains would pass without complaints or intervention. It was not unusual for Janice to call me at home for reassurance that a headache or indigestion that Jacob had been ignoring was unlikely to do him harm.

"Four days?" I asked in disbelief. "He's been sick for four days and you are just calling me now?"

"I know," Janice said in resignation, "but you know how he is.

He wouldn't let me call. I decided that I was going to call tonight as soon as he fell asleep. I'm sorry it's so late. I hope you are not in bed."

In fact, I had been in bed, but the sound of her voice jolted me awake instantly. It was an uneasy alertness. For Janice to call—and at this hour—Jacob must be seriously ill.

"I thought it was just the flu," she told me with a worried voice. "He was fine that morning but by the afternoon had a sore throat, horrible muscle aches, and a fever of 102. He has had a deep cough but only started to bring up a dark green sputum tonight. He is so weak. He hasn't eaten a thing since this started."

"Did he have a flu shot this year?" I started to ask before interrupting myself. "Never mind, I forgot who we were talking about. It certainly does sound like flu, at least at first. With the productive cough, though, I'm a little concerned about pneumonia. Is there any chance you can get him to the office in the morning?"

"There is no chance of that, doctor," she said. "He's going to be mad when he finds out that I called you tonight, but I don't care. I don't need his cooperation to call you. I'll never get him in the car against his will though. In case you haven't noticed, he's a very stubborn man."

With more than a little reluctance, I surrendered to the circumstances that no mortal could control and called in some antibiotics for Jacob to the all-night pharmacy near their home. Janice promised to call me immediately if he showed the slightest signs of getting worse and I resolved that I would go to Jacob if he wouldn't come to me. There were good reasons why I stopped making house calls years earlier, but for Jacob, there wouldn't be a moment's hesitation.

But it wouldn't be necessary. By the following afternoon, Jacob was already feeling better. His fever was down and his body aches were gone. He started to eat the next day; not much, but enough to make both Janice and I feel better.

The ring of the telephone again woke me from a sound sleep the following night and I knew before picking it up that it was about Jacob. Expecting to hear Janice's voice, the male voice on the line took me by surprise. It was the emergency room physician at the hospital. My relief was short-lived, however. He was calling about Jacob.

"He came in by squad," he said. "It sounds like his wife found him seizing. He doesn't look good. I'm concerned that he aspirated. We may need to put him on the ventilator."

My eyes fell on Janice the instant I rushed through the sliding doors of the emergency room. She stood leaning against the wall that led from the waiting room to the patient care area. I had never before seen the emotion that filled her eyes that night. She was terrified.

"They won't let me back with him," she sobbed. "Someone said he may not live. He was doing better, honestly he was. I left him for just a few minutes to go make some tea. He seemed nervous tonight and I thought it would help calm him down. When I went back in the bedroom, he was a horrible blue color and shaking all over. I don't think he was breathing when the rescue squad got there. Please, make them let me see him."

That Jacob didn't look good was an understatement. He looked horrible. The emergency room team was huddled around my friend. Despite the medication to silence his seizures, his body still trembled and his skin gave off a bluish cast. He did not respond to questions or seemed to notice the needles that pieced his skin to draw samples of blood. The monitor over his bed reported a rapid heart rate, high blood pressure, and despite the clear mask that covered his face, an oxygen level in his bloodstream that could not sustain life.

As I watched, an endotracheal tube was inserted into Jacob's trachea and he was connected to the ventilator. Anticonvulsants and increasingly larger doses of sedation were infused through his intravenous lines, but his tremors persisted.

"Is he a nice man?" the charge nurse asked me.

I nodded my head *yes*, understanding the inference she was making. Far too often, it seemed to be the exceptionally nice person that faired the worst in the emergency room.

Jacob was transferred to the intensive care unit where he would receive the best treatment modern medicine could provide. Unfortunately, we didn't know what we were treating. All of his laboratory studies came back normal. While the initial chest x-ray was good, we were concerned that Jacob had aspirated—gastric fluids being inhaled into the lungs and airways—during his seizure. Subsequent x-rays would be telling. For now, all we could do was provide the essentials of life and wait.

Although I tried, sleep eluded me during what was left of the night. I was frustrated and worried. I couldn't help Jacob if I didn't know what was wrong with him, and I didn't have a clue. The pulmonologist that I asked to see Jacob didn't fair much better. Follow-up chest x-rays indeed looked like aspiration pneumonia, and while it was a serious problem, it did not provide the answers I was looking for.

Janice was asleep in a chair next to Jacob's bed when I made rounds the following morning. A hospital blanket covered her, no doubt placed there by Jacob's nurse. I worked quietly and stepped softly so as not to wake her. I wasn't quite sure if my gesture was for her benefit or for mine. A sleeping wife cannot ask questions for which there are no answers.

"She hasn't been out of that chair all night," Jacob's nurse said. "I feel sorry for her. She said that the last time she left his bedside he ended up here."

There seems to be an unwritten law in medicine that long nights without sleep are followed by even longer days. My office staff had the uncanny ability to bring in those patients with the greatest needs on those days that I seemed to have the lowest capacity to give. The complaints of back pain, indigestion, and fatigue that filled my day seemed so trivial when I thought of Jacob lying in that hospital bed. Still, it was good to be busy.

Jacob's office chart sat on my desk and taunted me throughout the day. Between patients, I would find myself leafing through its pages, looking for answers when I wasn't even sure what the questions were. At day's end, I slipped the chart into my briefcase to take home with me. Perhaps I simply hadn't studied it enough.

I stopped by the hospital to see Jacob on my way home but he hadn't improved any during the day. In fact, he seemed a little worse to me. The ventilator was requiring higher pressures to breathe for Jacob and the concentration of oxygen that he needed was greater than it was in the morning. It was a combination I had seen before and it made me uneasy. Perhaps it was the look in Janice's face that unsettled me the most. Her eyes were red and swollen from crying and there was a look of surrender about her, as if the battle had already been lost.

Not having slept the night before, sleep should have come easy for me that night, but it didn't. I had had sick patients before, far too many of them, but I always seemed to know what was wrong with them even if I didn't know exactly how to help them. I knew none of those things with Jacob. It was a frightening uncertainty and uncommon dreams kept taking me back to an earlier place in an earlier time when I stood atop a tall ladder at the fire academy. The bitter taste in my mouth and the pounding in my chest I felt then was the same that plagued me now. I suspected there was a message buried deep within my awareness, but I was just too exhausted to see it.

I was filled with dread on my drive to the hospital the next morning. Most days found me irritated with slow traffic and frustrated by red lights that seemed specially programmed just to inconvenience me. On this day, I would have welcomed such delay, but the commute had never been easier or faster. Even the elevators in the hospital, typically the definition of wait and annoyance, whisked me instantly to the intensive care unit. There was a tear in my eye as I held the morning chest x-ray up to the light next to Jacob's bed. The pristine lucency that characterized his lungs just the day before had been replaced by dense white haze. The ventilator pressures and oxygen concentration had again been increased during the night. There could be no doubt. Jacob was in ARDS—adult respiratory distress syndrome—and it couldn't have been a bigger problem for him. I had seen it many times as a resident and many of those patients died. But Jacob was more than a patient as was the lady that sat by his side, and while I was determined to travel this journey with them, it just didn't seem to be enough.

Morning office hours passed in numbness and with a sadness that penetrated my soul. I longed for the peace and clarity of thought that I had always found in the woods of Demazie Hollow. It seemed so far away, yet the rustle of leaves and the song of birds that filled my thoughts spoke of a closeness that I always recognized, but perhaps never fully understood.

My lunch hour was spent on a courtyard bench not far from my office. I needed more than food that day and while I was not in the sanctuary of my woods, there were a few trees nearby. The song of the titmouse was replaced by the gentle purr of the pigeons that wandered about at my feet and the antics of the squirrels were performed by the toddler who found delight in a colony of ants harvesting breadcrumbs under the bench nearby. With closed eyes, I felt the sun warming my face and arms. Yes, there was peace here too.

An old man sat down clumsily at the end of my bench. He was tall and thin and the coarse features of his weathered face depicted a map of a difficult journey. He wore a long coat—one inappropriately heavy for the mild weather—with torn pockets and frayed edges. He looked hungry and I wondered when was the last time he had eaten. He clutched a small, brown paper bag that did little to conceal the bottle within. His hands were creased and darkened and trembled a bit. He seemed out of place here and I wondered if he too was searching for peace.

I could almost feel the breeze that winds its way through the rises and falls and the twists and turns of Demazie Hollow while sitting on that bench. I could almost smell the sweetness of the honeysuckle vine that weaves its way through the fabric of the woods there. I most certainly felt the stillness—the forgotten part of myself—that I had discovered there. Sitting on that bench in the middle of a big city didn't seem that much different from the large rock in the Hollow; it seemed impossible that there could be a problem without a solution.

With a start, I was instantly alert and jumped to my feet, startling the old man sharing my bench. That was it! That was the answer!

Running off toward my car, I stopped abruptly alongside a sidewalk vendor, my momentum nearly causing me to fall. Fishing in my pockets, I pulled out a ten-dollar bill and handed it to the vendor. "Would you do me a favor?" I asked. "Would you a make a couple of hot dogs and something to drink for that old man sitting over there?"

The startled lady looked at me a bit suspiciously then broke out in a smile that seemed too large for her face. "Of course I will, Mister," she beamed, "and aren't you special."

"No ma'am," I said hastily before running off, "he is."

Once in my car, I quickly pulled Jacob's office chart from my briefcase. I only needed a brief glance before setting it aside and speeding off toward the hospital. Janice jumped when I rushed into Jacob's room, his chart in hand.

"How much does he drink, Janice?" I asked quickly.

She seemed startled by the question and glanced at her adult son who was sitting next to her, Jacob's ventilator keeping rhythmic time in the background.

"A couple," she said with a shrug of her shoulders and a bewildered look on her face.

"No," I said holding up his file, "that's what it says in here, but I need to know more. Now, how much does he drink?"

"He has a couple of drinks with meals," she replied, now with a hint of defensiveness in her voice, "and maybe two or three before going to bed."

"What kind of drinks, how large are the glasses?" I pried.

"Only mixed drinks," she said. "The glasses are pretty big, but not all of that is liquor, you know."

"How many bottles do you go through in a week, Janice?" I asked softly.

She grew silent for a moment and looked over at her son as a tear fell from her cheek. It was only then that she seemed to grasp the significance of my questions. "Two or three," she said in a hushed voice, "some weeks four. But, doctor, he's a good man."

"I know he's a good man, Janice," I said as I placed my hand upon hers. "This has nothing to do with good or bad. When was his last drink?"

"Not since he's been sick," she said emphatically. "It's been a good week, so you see, it can't possibly have anything to do with him now."

When she saw the look in my face, she started to cry. It was not the look of a physician, but of an old friend. "It's bad, isn't it, Bill?" she asked.

"Yes, it's bad." I said. "Jacob is an alcoholic and he is going through alcohol withdrawal. Some call it DTs and as many as half of patients with this die. But Jacob has even greater problems. He has aspiration pneumonia and respiratory failure. He is very sick and I'm not sure he is going to survive this. But we know what we are treating now and that's a huge step forward. Whatever happens, we're going to face it together."

The days that followed were difficult ones—difficult for Jacob, his family, and his doctor. His lungs worsened daily until he reached the point that it was not possible for him to get any worse. Only then did he show a modicum of improvement. Maybe it wasn't improvement at all, but for those starved for good news, not getting any worse was a cause for celebration. While he could talk to us, the slowing of his heart rate and stabilization of his blood pressure indicated that the tremendous amount of medication used to treat his alcohol withdrawal was indeed helping. Through it all, Janice never left his bedside.

It was not until his tenth day in the intensive care unit that Jacob was well enough to be removed from the ventilator, but he was far from the Jacob I had known. While he was aware of activity around him, he was unable to respond to it. He couldn't walk and standing required the help of two physical therapists. He couldn't feed himself or drink from the water glass that always sat at his bedside. Still, his survival was nothing less than a miracle.

Jacob was transferred to the best rehabilitation hospital in the region. There life started over for him. He learned how to do everything all over again—from talking and walking to dressing and feeding himself. The gains achieved in rehabilitation, while dramatic, were far from enough to permit Jacob to return home and he required a prolonged stay in a nearby nursing home. Ever so gradually, Jacob became closer to the person he once was.

It was the better part of a year before I would see Jacob in the office again. I had never seen Janice happier. The physical therapy had gone well. From watching him walk to grasping my hand in greeting, I never would have known he had been so ill. But the body and mind heal in different ways and at different rates. His mind was still healing.

"How much do you remember, Jacob?" I asked during our office visit.

"The first thing I remember is waking up one morning at the rehab center," he said. "Everything before that is blank."

As they stood to leave, Jacob turned and faced me. "Do I know you, sir?" he asked.

"Yes," I replied, "we were old friends, and we will be again."

"He asked me the same thing," Janice said. "He had been home from the nursing home for several weeks when one night in bed he turned to me and asked, 'Do I know you?' I thought he had been acting unusually shy when I would put him in the shower every day. Poor guy, you have to wonder who he thought I was."

"I thought you were a very friendly nurse from the hospital," Jacob said.

Normally, I would have found such a story quite amusing, as I am sure Janice had intended, but I couldn't help but notice that Jacob was not smiling. The unease I saw in his eyes was heart wrenching and I struggled to comprehend just how difficult his journey these past months must have been for him. His friends and family had cheered his recovery, but they didn't understand that his struggle didn't start until he got well. I wasn't all that certain that Jacob believed Janice was indeed his wife.

As the months passed, the road upon which Jacob journeyed seemed to straighten and have fewer bumps and potholes. I would see Jacob every two weeks and with each visit, I could see improvement. Often the improvement was subtle, but there could be no mistake that it was there. It wasn't long before Jacob was puttering around in his shop. He didn't always understand why he was working on a project, but he followed the direction in which Janice pointed and allowed his soul to once again create beauty for others.

More than a year had passed when Jacob paused one day before leaving the examination room after one of his routine office appointments. Our visits had once again become warm and relaxed and I was surprised by the seriousness that I could see in his face. "Do you remember," he asked, "when I asked if I knew you and you told me that we had been old friends and would be again?"

"Sure I do, Jacob," I said.

"You were right," he said. "Thank you."

Life had pretty much returned to normal for Jacob and Janice. Business was good and their home was always filled with friends and family. Spoiling their grandchildren became their life's work. We seldom spoke of the earlier years, mainly because that Jacob no longer existed. Much of his memory returned, although the time he spent in the hospital and in rehabilitation were gone forever. Also gone was his desire for alcohol and, in fact, any recollection that he used to drink. It was one of the miracles of healing that I did not appreciate at the time.

But there would be reminders of that earlier life. The years of alcohol use had taken its toll and we would discover that Jacob had cirrhosis. It was a diagnosis that never seemed to bother either of them. He was alive and life was good.

It was the awareness of the cirrhosis, however, that prompted me to send Jacob to the hospital when Janice called one night to report that he was vomiting blood. It wasn't much blood, but the emergency room physician agreed that he should be watched in the hospital for a day or two. He was taken to endoscopy the following morning and large esophageal varices—enlarged veins within the esophagus that can bleed easily and severely—were discovered, no doubt a complication of the cirrhosis. Despite normal laboratory studies and complaints from Jacob, he was transferred to the Teaching Hospital where he was admitted to the intensive care unit.

As was typical, Jacob and Janice charmed the doctors and nurses at the Teaching Hospital. They liked the resident physician that was assigned to care for Jacob and noted that he looked so much like their eldest grandson. Somewhere amidst the talk of ballgame scores, golf, and refinishing coffee tables, the young physician apologetically informed Jacob that he needed to insert an intravenous line into a large vein in his chest. Even though Jacob was doing fine, it was a policy for ICU patients with esophageal varices to have a central line. It was a policy that the young doctor thought seriously about ignoring—it was a procedure that he hated to do to people—but there would be hell to pay on rounds the following morning if Jacob didn't have one.

Janice didn't mind spending a few minutes alone in the waiting room. She hated needles and by the sounds of this one, she wouldn't be very much support to Jacob if she remained in the room. As was often the case in the hospital, it took considerably more time preparing for a procedure than it actually took to perform it.

In mask, sterile gown, and gloves, Jacob's doctor took the surgical sponge saturated with antiseptic and scrubbed the skin of the right side of Jacob's neck and shoulder. He could feel Jacob tremble slightly beneath his touch. It made him feel bad. His patient had been so calm and relaxed earlier and he felt guilty about taking that away from him. As he prepared the site where he would insert the needle, he noticed a small drop of blood on Jacob's chin. It was so very small and as he leaned closer to get a better look, he saw a second drop trickle from Jacob's nose.

"How do you feel, Mr. Keller?" the young doctor asked.

Jack turned his head slightly and looked at his doctor. It was a look the young clinician had never seen before and it frightened him. Within seconds, the trickle of blood became a stream and flowed down Jacob's face. Jacob opened his mouth to speak, but instead of words came a fountain of blood. Calls for help were answered from every corner of the intensive care unit, but it was of little use. Within minutes, Jacob was gone.

As quickly as that room had filled with doctors and nurses responding to the crisis, it emptied, leaving Jacob's doctor standing in stunned shock next to his patient's bed. He took a few steps backward and sat down heavily on a stainless steel stool in the corner of the room. Blood still dripped from his hands. It had soaked through his gown and oozed from between the laces of his shoes. Dry blood had caked across the surface of his glasses, providing an even darker view of life at that moment.

An older nurse watched from the doorway. She had been caring for ICU patients—and the doctors that cared for them—since I was an intern. Her tough exterior softened and the practiced harshness in her eyes melted away as she approached the motionless doctor.

"I've got to go talk to Mrs. Keller," she heard him mumble.

"You are going to do no such thing," she said emphatically, peeling the bloodied latex gloves from his hands, "not looking like this. She is going to remember tonight the rest of her life. This shouldn't be part of her memories."

The well-schooled doctor looked more like a young boy as she loosened the ties on his gown. "First, we are getting you out of these clothes and then you are taking a long, hot shower in the call room. While you do that, I'll find you something to wear and make a pot of strong coffee. Then you will talk to Mrs. Keller."

Placing her hands on each side of his face, she peered into his eyes and said, "After that, you and I are going to sit down and have a good cry."

It was another late-night telephone call that brought word about Jacob. I recognized the woman's voice with the distinctive German accent immediately, although it was the first time she had ever called me. She had just sent Janice home with family, and while there was nothing I could do for them that night, she wondered if I would come to the hospital anyway. There was still someone there that might need help.

After a half-hour of looking, I found Michael Morten sitting on a bench outside the lobby of the Teaching Hospital. The hospital scrubs that he wore seemed inappropriate for the cool night air, but he didn't appear uncomfortable. The second-year medical resident gave me a quizzical look as I sat down next to him.

"I hear you've had quite a night, doctor," I said

"Good news travels fast," he replied with soft sarcasm. "I'll bet the parking attendant knows about the ICU doc that came unglued tonight. It's been two hours and my pager hasn't gone off once. That's never happened before. Even the ER must be afraid to call me."

He took a deep breath and looked up at the clear night sky. Even with the city lights, the brilliance of the heavens begged for attention. "Look at all the stars," he said with a touch of awe in his voice. "We forget how small we are. I thought I knew a lot of medicine. I thought I had seen it all. But I never knew someone could die that fast and that horribly. One minute we were talking about reupholstering chairs. A few minutes later, he was dead. He was such a nice man. You would have liked him."

"I know," I said softly, "and I did. Jacob was my patient for many years."

Even in the dimness of the streetlights, I could see Michael's eyes become misty. His lip quivered as he said, "I'm so very sorry. If I would have had the central line in earlier we might have been able to save him."

"Michael, look at me," I said, pausing until his eyes were focused on mine. "Even if you had that much blood just waiting to be transfused in his room, do you really believe you could have pushed it through IV tubing as fast as it was coming out of him? And how would you have stopped the bleeding? That would have been difficult on the operating table.

"Life can change in the blink of an eye and all of our training, technology, and even our conceit cannot alter that reality. More often than we would like to admit, we can be nothing more than spectators in our patients' lives, but if we open ourselves to that possibility, the journeys that we are privileged to observe are nothing less than miraculous. Maybe our role is not to change the journey but to be a witness to it. Maybe healing is helping others get the most out of their travel through life, no matter where it might lead."

"I certainly didn't help Mr. Keller," he said sadly.

"I'm not so sure, Michael," I insisted. "Jacob loved nothing more than talking about his work. Sharing something that you love with others and taking delight in that sharing is not a bad way to spend your final hour of life. He was a quiet and private man and I know that he would have been very frightened in the ICU. You spared him that.

"The longer I do this work the more I am convinced there are no accidents. There was a reason for you to be at Jacob's side tonight, if not for him, then maybe for his wife. I understand you were very good with her."

"I sure wasn't very professional," he said, sounding embarrassed. "I cried like a baby."

"I wonder from where the notion came," I thought out loud, "that doctors shouldn't feel, and if they find themselves doing so they must never show it, particularly to their patients. There are times in medicine, quite often actually, when our science is not enough, when all that we have to offer is ourselves. Tonight was one of those nights. Jacob Keller was in the finest intensive care unit in the city, yet he died. But for the compassion of a young doctor, one willing to share his humanity, Janice Keller would never know that her husband died in caring hands. In your face, she could see how special he was. That knowledge will be very comforting to her in the days to come; it will help her heal."

We sat together in silence, gazing off into the night sky for several minutes before Michael looked at me curiously and asked, "You didn't come in for Mr. Keller, did you, sir? You didn't know he was here. Katarina called you, didn't she?"

I smiled broadly at his deduction.

"I used to think she was a witch," he said in obvious discomfort. "I never really saw her before tonight. She spent over an hour cleaning up Mr. Keller before she would let his wife see him. She certainly didn't have the time to do that—the unit was very busy."

"And what she did for me," he said with a breaking voice before looking away.

"Michael," I said, "you are going to look back on tonight as one of the most difficult nights of your career. But I've had the incredible fortune of special teachers in my life that helped me discover the astonishing potential that hides in dark times—wisdom that would otherwise elude us, the opportunity to serve, and an understanding that the good times will be all the better because of it. If we are open to the possibility and have the courage to embrace the hard times for what they might teach us, we will discover the special teachers there to help us. Jacob, Janice, and especially Katarina, if you let them, can be your teachers. If you do, tonight will become the awareness that you are so much more than your training and the expectations of others, perhaps it will be the first time that you discovered healing."

It would be several days before Janice stopped by the office to talk about Jacob. I was unaccustomed to seeing her without him and perhaps for the first time I could see the fascinating uniqueness that was her soul. She seemed very much at peace, something that surprised me, and I told her so.

"It was a tremendous shock," she said, "but as horrible as the experience was at the hospital, it helped me. After all we had gone through, the possibility that Jacob could die that night hadn't crossed my mind. When that young doctor came out to talk to me, I knew the instant I looked at his face. I don't think the possibility that Jacob could die had crossed his mind either. Being there at the hospital helped because it was obvious nothing could have been done. It was his time. I'm thankful it didn't happen at home. He spared me that.

"At first I was so angry. I had just gotten Jacob back only to have him taken away again. It didn't seem fair. Being alone that first night at home, I remembered what it was like the time before when he got sick. Everywhere I looked, I saw a reminder of us together, some from our life many years ago but many things from the last couple of years. I suddenly felt very special and very blessed. The two of us; we fell in love all over again. People often wonder if they had something to do over again, would they. I don't have to wonder; I lived it and it was wonderful.

"The past year couldn't have been more special. We were each other's first love and we lived it twice. When you know what mistakes to avoid from the first time around, all that is left is bliss. That did not die with Jacob. That will live within me forever. It is a gift that would not have been possible had it not been for those dark days when Jacob first got sick. It is a gift that would not have been possible had it not been for a special doctor that walked those dark days with us."

With a hug, a whispered thank you, and a tear in her eye, Janice left my office that day. Her tears were not of sadness but of overwhelming gratitude for a journey that was made better by sharing it with others. Along the journey, there was wisdom discovered through darkness, great beauty seen in chaos, and doctors learning how to heal.

CHAPTER 9

Innocence Lost

*I have learned silence from the talkative, tolerance
from the intolerant, and kindness from the unkind.
I should not be ungrateful to those teachers.*

KAHLIL GIBRAN

*Every great and deep difficulty bears in itself its own solutions.
It forces us to change our thinking in order to find it.*

NIELS BOHR

I had seen those eyes before, and the look frightened me. They were
tired, but it was more than that. They were harried, but it was
worse than that. They were confused, but there was still more. They
were needy, but there was yet a deeper message. It was the same look
that I had seen in Sam's eyes, but she had hidden it better. In fact, it
was the same look I had been seeing in the eyes of young doctors for
many years—the better trained, the better they were at concealing
it, until its origins simply faded away into the unconsciousness we
call professionalism.

Realizing that his empty gaze had lingered in my direction far too long, the medical student sitting across from me in the nursing station looked away with a startled jump, but not before reaching deep into my soul and touching me. It was late morning and the medical teams were completing morning rounds. The nursing station filled rapidly with residents and students focused on their assigned tasks. There were progress notes to write, orders to enter, consultations to request, and discharges to arrange. Somewhere in the process, there would be learning.

With an unsettling chill, I remembered the first time I had seen those eyes. It was so many years ago, yet the vividness and suddenness of the recollection told me it had been only a moment ago. They peered back at me from a mirror in a Texas motel room. They peered from a soul wandering in darkness, looking for hope, and desperate for purpose.

Memories from medical school seldom visited me and it was curious they would do so at that time, particularly memories from a brief and difficult period in what was otherwise a very positive experience. Among the curriculum of medical school are buried subtle lessons that have little to do with caring for patients. Embracing tradition and the ways of the past, mastering the clinical mystique, and learning how to *play the game* are ever present in medical education. It was *playing the game* that took me to Texas.

The pressure to select a specialty haunts medical students from their earliest days and influences the course work they select and the timing in which they take it. Clinical rotations provide more than experience in patient care; they can yield letters of recommendation necessary in landing residency positions after graduation. Acceptance into competitive residency programs can be enhanced when students spend a month or two of their training at the desired institution. It was a pursuit that would profoundly change me.

August of my senior year in medical school found me in a strange place, far from my home and the comfort of familiarity and routine. The Texas Medical Center in Houston boasted of the best health care in the world. The opportunity to train there was an extraordinary one, if not an intimidating one. I would spend the month at one of the many teaching hospitals as an acting intern, perhaps the most challenging and difficult rotation of medical school. To do so alone, far from the support of family and friends, seemed a better idea months earlier than it did on the day I first drove into that city.

Home was to be an aging motel, not far from the Astrodome. The rooms were small, dark, and worn, but the price was affordable. The motel catered to patients and visitors of the medical center, providing kitchen facilities and a lounge for families. The buildings of the motel surrounded a courtyard dominated by a fenced and locked swimming pool, drained and abandoned many years earlier. Pockets of lush green plantings dotted the courtyard, perhaps the remnants of a better time, but nonetheless, a testimony that caring hands and hearts must be nearby.

The parking lot, deeply scarred with cracks and potholes, was filled with an eclectic collection of automobiles that had seen better days. License plates from across the country spoke of long journeys and the search for hope. It seemed a fitting place to park my own car, an aging Chevy that had faithfully made the quest from Ohio. It would be my first extended stay away from home, and I missed it already.

The aroma that filled the hallways of that motel, however, would carve the deepest impression into my memories. There was staleness mixed with a medicinal smell and just a touch of antiseptic. It was strangely clinical and filled the air with a tinge of sadness that I did not understand. As floorboards creaked beneath my feet, I wondered about each wooden door as I passed and what stories must lay behind their darkened frames and peeling paint. I wondered too what stories would soon lay behind my own door just a few more steps away.

At 6 am, it was already eighty degrees when I walked toward the teaching hospital for the first time. A heavy haze clung to the tops of trees and the hospital seemed to rise up from a mystical foundation. It was huge, much larger than any of our hospitals back home. People flowed through every door like bees swarming about their hive as ambulances waited their turn for an open bay at the emergency entrance. The scope of the early morning activity surprised me and I walked through those doors for the first time with more than a little apprehension.

The lobby was cavernous and looked more fitting for a warehouse than a hospital. People were everywhere—many had obviously spent the night there. The initial impression of bedlam softened a bit after many moments of shocked scrutiny, no doubt, with mouth agape. If it was bedlam, than it was a controlled bedlam. Everyone seemed to move with purpose, or at least with practiced determination.

I had been instructed to take the north elevators to the twelfth floor medical ward. There I would meet my team. Four banks of elevators served the lobby and impressive crowds gathered around each. It would be many minutes of waiting before I would find myself wedged into the corner of an elevator that belonged to an earlier time. It shuddered and inched slowly upward, as I silently estimated the weight of my companions and glanced nervously at the maximum-capacity sign. The doors opened at every floor and with every lurch upward, my apprehension grew.

"My God!" I whispered softly to myself as I stepped off the elevator. Nothing could have prepared me for what I saw. The twelfth-floor medical ward was just that—a huge room with over a hundred beds. It was as if I was looking at a photograph of a nineteenth-century hospital ward, except, of course, I wasn't supposed to be in the picture. I stood in disbelief while studying the scene before me. Perhaps this was all a dream and I would soon awaken back in my motel room, no doubt in a cold sweat. But it was no dream.

The room was filled with row after row of hospital beds, each separated by a movable screen on wheels. Beside each bed sat a nightstand and a straight-back chair. On each nightstand was a reading lamp. The north half of the room was reserved for female patients while *12 South* tended to the men. Nursing stations were strategically placed around the periphery of the room, one station for every two or three rows of beds. Three of the four walls were of large windows that opened to the Houston air. Large fans hung suspended from the ceiling, but still it felt uncomfortably warm.

A smiling face and insistent voice brought me back to reality. It was a place that I wasn't sure I wanted to be. "You must be the new guy," the voice said. "I'm Ben. Don't look so worried, you are going to be fine. Let's go meet the boss."

Ben was also a senior medical student and would be serving as an acting intern with me. There would be four of us on the team as well as four interns. Each intern would have a junior medical student to supervise. It was a much larger ward team than I had been used to at home, no doubt an indication of the volume of patients that we would be caring for. The awesome responsibility of supervising such a large team was not lost on me and I already felt a deep respect for the senior resident that I had yet to meet.

Doug Sanchez was that resident and he barely looked up from his work when Ben introduced me to him. "You can call me Doug," he said curtly. "Lose the shirt and tie. We just wear scrubs around here. You can pick them up in the laundry department in the basement. You'll go through a couple pairs a day when it gets busy, so get plenty.

"I just have one rule," he said. "Don't kill anyone! You had better know what you're doing because I don't have time to teach you. After you work up a patient, tell me what you are going to do, don't ask me what to do.

"You have a new patient in the ER to admit. You have one hour to turn in admission orders and two hours to get a note on the chart. When you are done with that, you have four old patients from last month's team to pick up. Rounds are at seven in the morning and we round with the attending at eight. Make sure you are prepared."

With that, my orientation to the teaching hospital was over. It was not the introduction that I had hoped for. My hands trembled slightly as I recorded the names of my new patients. My mouth was dry and there was a fullness in my throat. They were subtle signs, easy to ignore and dismiss, but I could not. I had experienced them before. It had been many years since fear had visited me so intimately. It was at the fire academy just before entering that burning house. Fear can be a useful tool in the fire service—it can save your life. But how could it serve me in this place? What did it have to do with healing?

Ben rode down with me in the elevator on the way to the emergency room. My new colleagues thought it best that I not go alone on my first visit. It would be a prudent gesture, one that would be greatly appreciated. For the third time in as many hours, I stood in shocked silence, this time in the main entrance to the emergency department. Like everything else at the teaching hospital, it was huge.

It was actually two emergency departments in one, one for medical problems and the other for surgical issues, each many times larger than the emergency room I was used to back home. A long corridor led to a triage desk where a nurse sat. Medical patients were directed to the right and surgical patients to the left. The corridor was filled with people lined in wait. I stared in disbelief at a young man leaning against a wall, his hands grasping his left side and his shirt saturated in blood. Ben barely raised an eyebrow.

My patient would be found in the respiratory treatment room along with a dozen other patients inhaling aerosolized medication deep into their lungs. I breathed a sigh of relief upon learning that he would be admitted for an asthma exacerbation—it was a problem that I was familiar with. My ease was short-lived, however. He spoke no English, and I, no Spanish. It was only then that I realized that much of the chatter that had surrounded me that morning was in Spanish. The tightness in my throat returned.

I would be the only member of the team that could not speak any Spanish, clearly a liability at a hospital serving Houston's disadvantaged neighborhoods. In keeping with the challenges of the day, none of the patients that waited for me upstairs would speak English.

I couldn't believe my eyes. It was Marty Drier, I was sure of it. I hadn't expected to meet anyone I knew in Texas, let alone someone from my own medical school. But there he was standing in the doorway of the auditorium. Noon conference was the major teaching activity for the Department of Medicine and attendance was expected of all. The auditorium started to fill some twenty minutes early each day, many bringing lunch with them. It was a large training program and every available seat would be taken. I was excited beyond belief at seeing Marty. Suddenly, I felt less alone.

Marty turned toward me when I shouted his name. Staring blankly in my direction, he didn't seem to know me. He looked horrible. His hair was a mess, his scrubs stained, and it looked like he had been sleeping in his lab coat. There was a momentary flash of recognition in his eyes, which quickly changed to a look of shock and confusion. I thought he was about to say something, but with the slightest shake of his head, he turned and melted into the auditorium. Perhaps I had made a mistake and it wasn't Marty after all.

Marty Drier was a favorite son at my medical school. One year my senior, he had graduated just several months earlier. He was the definition of success and potential. If anyone would rise to greatness, there was no doubt he would head the list. His father was on the faculty as a professor of medicine and was more feared than respected among my colleagues. He was ruthless in his expectations of others and I often wondered what it was like for Marty living in his very big shadow.

If I had any doubts that the resident I had seen was Marty, unfortunately, they would be quickly dispelled. Dr. Drier was called upon to present one of his patients to the conference. Standing at the podium, he looked like a deer in headlights. He appeared weak and timid and his voice was barely audible. He presented a middle-aged man that was admitted the day before with a lung mass. His performance was disorganized, tentative, and painful to watch. Clearly, Marty wasn't prepared. Sensing weakness, the predators in the room circled for the attack.

The faculty pounced first, questioning the accuracy of his history and physical examination findings. The senior residents criticized his diagnoses while his fellow interns found fault with his management decisions. Even medical students stood to voice doubt and concern.

It was a grilling unprecedented in my experience and I sat in the back of the auditorium wide-eyed, the tightness in my throat once again my companion. The room tingled with excitement and you could feel the energy in the air. But it was an energy void of learning, of compassion, and of healing.

Late that night, I received an unexpected page to the residents' call room. I was still in the hospital learning about my patients. Our first attending rounds were in the morning and I wanted to be prepared. Sitting in the corner of a darkened call room, I found Marty waiting for me.

"Please don't tell them about me," he said in a pleading voice. "Please don't tell them about my father."

His voice cracked with emotion—emotion that seemed foreign to the Drier name. There were tears in his eyes. Indeed, I had been mistaken. This was not the Marty Drier I had known. It was someone else. Gone was the confidence, the vision, and even the touch of arrogance that had once defined him. The transformation and rapidity with which it had overcome him were deeply troubling to me. While we had never been close, I was filled with worry for him. He had lost weight and I wondered when the last time he had slept was. The energy of the sadness that filled his soul reached out and touched mine and I became filled with worry for myself. He represented the best and the brightest—what chance would I have?

Ronald Presley Harley III, M.D. was embroidered in red above the left breast pocket of his pristine white lab coat. Crisply starched and pressed, the coat was buttoned from top to bottom and reminded me of a tortoise's protective shell. He stood erect and walked with a slow, almost practiced gait that would be expected of a military commander. While not much older than the rest of us, it appeared that he very much wanted to be. He would be our attending for the month.

"Mr. Hernandez came to the ER with symptoms of a heart attack," I said in presenting my first patient during attending rounds.

"And what was his heart attacking him with?" interrupted Dr. Harley.

"I'm sorry, sir?" I asked, not expecting to be interrupted so early in my presentation.

"Hearts don't attack people," he replied, making no effort to hide the disgust in his voice. "Doctors call it *myocardial infarction*. You may not understand it or have a clue what to do about it, but at the very least you should be able to talk like a doctor."

"I'm sorry," I said, "I thought it was proper to relate the *chief complaint* in the words of the patient."

"Not if it makes us sound stupid." He snorted. "Would you come to rounds screaming if you were presenting a patient in labor? Impression is everything in medicine. You always have to look and sound like professionals."

Nothing in my presentation met with his approval as evidenced by the frequent interruptions and observations on how *good doctors* would do things differently. What little self-confidence had survived to that point was slowly leaking from my being. I was both frustrated and intimidated. To my great relief, my colleagues faired little better during their presentations. Perhaps it wasn't just me.

Rounds lasted three hours that first morning. With the amount of work we had to do, it seemed too great of a price to pay for what we had received in return. Clearly, learning to care for patients would have to come from some other place. I had no idea where that place might be.

I joined Ben in the cafeteria later that day. He looked as tired as I felt and it was only the second day of the rotation. The cafeteria was immense—the dining area easily accommodating several hundred people. It was an environment that should have been filled with laughter and high spirits, but curiously, there was none. Aimlessly gazing across the room, the realization first came to me—I hadn't seen anyone smile at the teaching hospital. No one looked happy.

As if aware of my thoughts, Ben looked up at me, shook his head, and said, "It's going to be a long month. In our medical school, we have to do this. Why are you here?" It was a question for which I had no answer.

It was Sunday, typically a short day in the hospital, and I made it back to my motel room before dark. It seemed so much more inviting than it did a couple of days earlier. That's when I saw those eyes looking back at me from the mirror. They were both familiar and strange. The strangeness startled me—I thought I knew that soul so well, but yet there was a darkness that I had not been aware of, a path that needed exploration.

Images of Marty haunted me. What were the odds of finding him in this place? Would I too fight the demons that seemed to posses him—not feeling smart enough, strong enough, hungry enough, or dedicated enough? I contemplated leaving, but where would my letter of recommendations come from? Where would I learn medicine?

A loaf of bread and a jar of peanut butter can sustain a medical student for many a day, but that night it was more than sustenance, it was a gourmet meal. It was a meal too precious for indoors and I wandered about the courtyard searching for a spot where I might sit and eat. At the end of the complex, off the cement walkway and tucked snugly between two buildings, there was an area that seemed out of place, perhaps forgotten. It was a small pocket of emerald opulence.

Oakleaf hydrangeas lined the walls of the adjacent buildings, the huge leaves providing the illusion of sitting in an oak woodlot back home, save for the abundant, cream-colored blossoms. An inviting bench had been placed among fronds of cinnamon and wood ferns and begged for careful, deliberate steps to reach it. Black-eyed susans and black-foot daisies filled in the voids with brilliant bursts of color. It seemed so late in the year for them to be blooming. Perhaps they had waited for me.

An old birdbath in need of repair sat among the ferns, its sides chipped and stained. Water dripped into it from a rusted pipe and provided an occasional note to the symphony of silence that enveloped me there. It seemed an unlikely paradox—a place so small that it seemed to stretch on forever—all the way home.

A whistled *peter-peter-peter* seemed to call from my past as a tufted titmouse revealed itself from behind a hydrangea leaf. I watched with fascination and awe as its curiosity brought it closer and closer to my resting place, much as I had watched as a boy when we first met. With tilted head it watched me, like a concerned friend from home, its crest rising and falling in emphasis. With all that had troubled my spirit in recent days, it was strange that tears would only now fill my eyes.

I sat oblivious of time as day slipped from the sky. I could not force myself to leave, profoundly touched by warmth that I sought to understand. In that inexplicable contentment, I became aware of another paradox. I came to this place seeking knowledge, but knew I would find something more. I came seeking advantage, but somehow I knew that the seeking was to be the advantage.

Hard work and long hours proved an excellent elixir for the discomfort of the initial days of my acting internship. It wasn't a cure, but it was effective treatment, even if the medicine did taste rather bitter. The language barrier made the struggle particularly difficult. My first week at the teaching hospital passed without being assigned a single patient that spoke English. I sensed conspiracy, particularly when all of the other students had received English-speaking patients. When I asked the senior resident about it one morning, he laughed saying, "Don't you see, it's a gift! Look how much time you save by not having to talk to patients. There's nothing they can tell you that you won't discover on labs or diagnostic studies."

In a few days time, I had had a crash course in Spanish and learned enough phrases that would help me pick up on major problems. But I had wanted more. How could we help if we did not understand? Understanding, my colleagues would remind me, was irrelevant to cure. Juanita helped me to see that, indeed, there was more.

I met Juanita in the throws of the emergency room's most hectic period, not that there was ever a quiet time there. Several hours of each day, typically in the late evenings, the controlled chaos of that space teetered precariously on the precipice of abandoned anarchy. The precision choreography of doctors, nurses, and ancillary support faltered somewhat, making it harder to find help with patients in all but the most urgent of circumstances. I found Juanita sitting on a stretcher in the middle of that turmoil, arms embracing her abdomen, rocking gently back and forth.

Naturally, she spoke no English, but it didn't require a translator to see that she was quite ill. Her skin was drawn and dry and the muscles of her face and arms had withered from their normal state of health. Despite her distended abdomen, she had obviously lost weight. Her eyes were deeply yellowed, but through their distress, I could see a kind and gentle soul. I knew nothing about this lady, but yet I liked her instantly. A woman stood by her side. From the resemblance, her age, and her worried look, I guessed her to be a sister.

"*Dolar*?" I asked.

She nodded yes and managed a smile that was uncharacteristically warm. It was a stupid question. Of course she was in pain. I had better questions, but didn't know how to ask them. After a frustrating search for help, I returned to Juanita's bedside with an orderly that was able to translate for me, but her sister was already gone.

I asked my questions and learned that he had been in pain for two, maybe three months. When I wanted to know why she waited so long before seeking help, the answer was short and simple. She had no money.

"Where's her sister?" I asked the orderly.

It seemed too simple a question to have driven the prolonged back and forth between my patient and the orderly. "She says she doesn't know, doc," the young man said, "but I don't believe her. I suspect they are undocumented. I'll bet you never see her face again."

The orderly was right, I never saw Juanita's sister again, or any visitor for that matter. Whatever might lay ahead for this lady, she would have to endure it alone. It seemed a cruel reality.

Language would be an effective, if not insurmountable, barrier to learning about Juanita. I cringed at the thought that my colleagues might be right, that all I would need to know to be able to care for her would come from lab and test results. And those results were not good. The bilirubin in her blood was very high and her kidney function was poor.

I learned early in medical school that you never wanted to become an interesting case at a teaching hospital. Juanita had become just that. The team hung on my every word as I presented Juanita the following morning in attending rounds. "What is your impression, *Doctor*?" Dr. Harley asked with a tinge of sarcasm in his voice.

"My impression is that of obstructive jaundice and renal failure," I answered without hesitation. "I suspect the renal failure is due to dehydration and should improve with IV fluids. We will need imaging to determine the cause of the obstructive jaundice."

While stroking his chin as if deep in thought, the attending paced the floor of the conference room for a full minute before stopping abruptly, turning to the senior resident and saying, "I agree. See to it." His lack of criticism seemed almost glowing praise and my colleagues exchanged looks of surprise. It was a happening that just days earlier would have brought me ecstasy, but something was different. I wanted more than to be right. Juanita needed more.

I wheeled Juanita down to ultrasound that evening, having convinced a technician to stay late in order to look at her gallbladder. I was hoping to find gallstones and the possibility that one was blocking the flow of bile from the gallbladder. There were other possibilities for the jaundice, of course, but they seemed too horrible to think about. Despite multiple attempts in various positions, the technician couldn't image the gallbladder well enough to aid in the diagnosis. Juanita would need a CT scan, but it would be many days before her kidneys would be healthy enough to tolerate the medication given during the scan. So we would wait, with those other possibilities not far from our thoughts.

"Rosario," Juanita would say to me every morning and I would shrug my shoulders in frustration. It didn't seem to be a question, but yet it was more than a statement. It was almost a plea that I didn't understand. I would see Juanita several times each day. The medication I prescribed eased her pain and the IV fluids slowly restored brightness to her eyes, but she had greater needs that troubled me. Each day I would bring her a Spanish-language newspaper, magazine, or book to read, or something small from the gift shop, and while she was thrilled by the gesture, they came far from filling that void.

The busy ward service made it difficult to spend much time with Juanita, but those visits seemed to bring her relief and calm, something that my medications were incapable of. Each night I would sit at her bedside and write my daily notes in the stack of charts that I brought with me. Unable to converse, we sat in silence. It was in that silence that I started to understand Juanita the best.

Juanita's CT of the abdomen was eventually obtained and revealed that which I had feared. The duration of her pain, the anemia, and the weight loss had made other possibilities unlikely, but until the final test results are in, denial can be your friend. Juanita had pancreatic cancer. The tumor was quite large and had already invaded surrounding organs. Medical school had taught me the grim survival statistics and I realized that most of that time had probably already been lived at home and in pain.

Ben joined me for lunch that day and our conversation turned to Juanita's test results. The entire team had suspected cancer by that time. "I wish I could find her sister," I commented between sips of coffee. "I think her name is Rose, she keeps asking for *Rosario*."

"Are you sure you have that word right?" Ben asked in surprise.

"I think so, why?" I replied.

"Well, *rosario* means rosary. Do you think she's catholic?" he pondered.

I was shaken by the revelation and embarrassed by its simplicity. Could this be the need I had felt her soul cry out for?

I quickly finished my work and left the hospital earlier than usual that day. With every trip to and from the hospital that month, I had driven by a small, yet stately catholic church. Soon I was climbing the sanctuary's steps but the door marked *church office* was locked. Disappointed, I looked at my watch and realized that while it was early for me, it was well past typical business hours. Turning to leave, I noticed a man working in a flower garden alongside the sanctuary. He smiled when I approached, set aside his tools, and stood to greet me. He was an older man with gray hair and was covered in dirt from head to toe.

"Everyone is gone for the day," he confirmed. "But I can call someone if it is important."

I thanked him for the offer but explained that I just wanted to know where I could buy a rosary. His quizzical look made me smile and I explained that I was working at the teaching hospital and had a patient that I was having trouble communicating with. "I'm not certain, but I believe she wants a rosary and I would like to get her one," I said.

The old man looked thoughtful for a moment and said, "Wait here a minute. I have a key and know where the secretary keeps a supply."

Not pausing to listen to my objections, he turned and quickly disappeared around the corner. He wasn't gone more than a minute when he returned holding a clear plastic envelope in his dirty hand. Inside was a string of beads and a crucifix. My hand trembled slightly taking the envelope from him and I was filled with incredible excitement. I was part of something extraordinary, although I didn't understand what that might be.

The gardener refused my offer of money, telling me that he had some pull with the secretary and would square things with her in the morning. Writing my name and hospital pager number on a peace of paper, I extracted a promise from him that the secretary would call me if I owed them any money. Placing the paper in his pocket, he returned to his flowers and I returned to the hospital. I was grateful to see that Juanita was sleeping when I approached her bedside that evening, but even in sleep, she did not seem at peace. I would not wake her. She would have a difficult day tomorrow and needed her rest. I gently pressed the rosary into her palm and quietly slipped away.

Cup of coffee in hand, I sat in the conference room reviewing my patients' laboratory results before making morning rounds. It was the way I started every day and I was finding some comfort in the routine. Juanita's labs looked horrible. I had had hopes that she was getting better, at least before I saw the CT scan the day before. Perhaps my colleagues had been right all along. The tools of medical technology have made the role of the patient almost irrelevant.

Juanita's kidney function was again worsening, she was severely anemic, and now her liver was failing. I had seen patients far more ill as a medical student, but that was in the role of an observer. It felt different being responsible for someone's care, even if that responsibility was a supervised one. It was a piercing defeat, not like that of a lost job, a failing grade, or being bested by a rival. This one soaked to the depth of my being—even my soul hurt. I could not offer her cure.

When the team stopped by Juanita's beside on rounds, we all looked a little surprised. Juanita was sitting up and greeted our approach with a broad smile. She had combed her hair and was wearing a hospital-issued robe over her gown. Obviously, she hadn't seen her test results that morning. The senior resident asked her about her pain in fluent Spanish. She told him that her pain was gone. Perhaps in disbelief, he pressed gently on her abdomen, but still she denied discomfort.

"What did you do to her?" he asked me as we stepped back from her bed. He seemed surprised and even a little irritated.

"Nothing," I said. "The nurse told me she hasn't requested any pain medication since last night."

"Have you told her yet?" he asked.

"No," I replied. "I've scheduled a medical translator to help me this morning. I'll talk to her about hospice and make arrangements to transfer her as soon as possible."

"Good," he said. Either he was oblivious to the obvious sadness in my voice, or he simply did not care. I didn't know which possibility disappointed me the most. "You need to spend your time with those that you can help."

I paused briefly to smile at Juanita as the rest of the team continued down the long row of beds. It was the best I had seen her since her admission and it made me happy, despite the knowledge of the heavy duty that awaited me later that morning. As I turned to leave, I noticed the rosary held gently in her hand.

The rosary was still in that hand when I sat beside Juanita later that morning, a medical translator standing behind me. She looked quizzically at the stranger that had intruded upon the silence we had grown accustomed to. Like a bolt of lightening came the realization that words are not necessary for communication. Perhaps they even hinder it.

"When am I going to die?" Juanita asked.

"Soon, I believe, Juanita," I replied with directness that I wouldn't have thought possible, "but I do not have the wisdom to answer that question. How did you know?"

"I've known since I got here," she said. "I see it in your eyes and feel it in your heart. It terrified me at first, but not now. An angel came to me last night and told me all about it. He told me that I wouldn't be alone and described the wondrous journey that awaits me." Juanita held open her outstretched hand to reveal the rosary. It glistened with a brilliance that I did not notice the previous day. "He left me this," she said.

Arrangements were made to transfer Juanita to hospice the following morning. The attending disapproved of my leaving rounds early to see her off, but strangely, I didn't care. A tall man dressed in a black suit was standing by Juanita's bed when I approached. He seemed to sense my presence and turned to face me.

"Good morning, doctor," he said in a booming voice with an outstretched hand.

He wore the collar of a Roman Catholic priest. "I'm not a doctor, sir," I said.

"And I'm not a gardener," he said with a warm smile, "but I do so love growing flowers. It's where I feel the closest to God."

I knew that face and the gray hair, but gone were the coveralls, the stooped posture, and the dirt. It was the gardener who had given me the rosary two days before.

"You don't have to worry about Juanita," he said softly. "She is going to stay at one of our facilities and members of the parish will visit every day. She will never be alone.

With tears in my eyes, I watched as the transporters moved Juanita to an ambulance stretcher. As they started to roll her away, she stopped them. Reaching out to me, she placed a hand on each side of my face and stared intently into my eyes. With a gentle kiss upon my forehead she said, "*Dios te bendiga.*"

When she had been rolled out of sight, the priest placed a hand on my shoulder and in a hushed voice said, "It means *God Bless You*, son. And He has—with the gift of healing. And He blessed Juanita by bringing you to this place. She came seeking cure, but instead found something much more precious—she found healing. It is not found through medicines, technology, or the expectations of doctors. It's found by those willing to consider another path and to be open to the wonders that they can hear in silence. You can hear that silence, son, and someday you will understand it. But you don't have to understand a gift to be able to use it.

"It's no accident that you are here. The answers you seek can be found in that silence that you hear so well, and that you shared with Juanita. Go to the special place where you hear it the best. It is a sacred place. For me, that quiet voice speaks the loudest in my garden. The answers will come.

"*Dios te bendiga,*" he said with a warm smile before turning and walking out of my life.

The fern fronds gently rose and fell like waves traveling across a lake, while the heads of daisies nodded approvingly in the evening air. He was right; this was a sacred place. Many an evening and early morning I had spent here, seeking answers when I didn't even know the questions. Instead, I found peace and the awareness that the importance of the journey was at least as great as that of the destination. Every step was to be cherished, honored, and squeezed for every drop of understanding it possessed.

The miraculous seemed common here, almost expected. I had thought the priest's visit to Juanita was miraculous, but as I reflected upon it, I realized that it had been no miracle. The priest did not come for Juanita; he had come for me. That was the miracle. Indeed, that quiet voice he spoke of seems so clear here. The titmouse, my friend from home, again danced among the hydrangeas, reminding me of a special place that awaited return. But the emerald greens, the blossoms of color, and even that titmouse are but a thought away, creating a special place within that I could visit at any time. Perhaps this was the understanding that he promised.

As the final traces of sunset disappeared from the sky, the heavens became alive with light from distant worlds. It was an unusually clear night and the multitude of stars was extraordinary. My attention was drawn to Polaris and the constellations of the north. Tomorrow they would lead me home, my stay here complete. I came seeking knowledge, but would leave with wisdom that would take years for me to understand. I found adversity an unlikely teacher, not to be avoided, but embraced. I discovered that our best teachers can be those who demonstrate paths upon which we should not take and encountered the unhappiness that spawns in journeys undertaken not for ourselves, but for the satisfaction of others. I experienced the power of silence and the irrelevance of words to the understanding of another. Perhaps for the first time, I realized there was a difference between curing and healing and that the difference was profound.

The pager on my belt pierced the silence like a knife. With irritation, I looked at the display. It was my office. I was home again at the Teaching Hospital. I had forgotten those earlier teachers, but not their lessons, many of which only now I have come to understand. The medical student was still there, the pain and confusion of the nursing station swirling about him. I walked across the room and sat next to him.

"Excuse me," I said, "but you look like someone with a problem.

Is there anything I can do to help?"

Surprised, and more than a little embarrassed, he shook his head slowly and said, "No, it's just this patient of mine. She has cancer and is not going to get better. I want so much to help her, but I don't know what to do."

"I had a patient like that when I was a medical student," I said. "Her name was Juanita; let me tell you about her."

CHAPTER 10

Silent Miracles

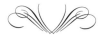

Let us be silent that we may hear the whispers of God

RALPH WALDO EMERSON

There are only two ways to live your life. One is as though nothing is a miracle. The other is as though everything is a miracle. I choose the latter.

ALBERT EINSTEIN

"Miracles just don't happen in medicine," I heard him say as the young-looking attending physician sat down with a small group of residents and students at the table next to me in the coffee shop. Ben Marsh was one of our junior faculty members at the Teaching Hospital, but he was clearly on the fast track for a leadership position in the department. He always thrilled in asking his team to join him for coffee after rounds and judging by the faces of those that surrounded him, there were other places they would rather have been. One of those faces belonged to Samantha and she gave me a wary smile as she took a seat across from her attending.

"Miracles just don't happen," he said again. "All I'm saying is that lady you presented on rounds this morning couldn't possibly have had pancreatic cancer. She was either mistaken about the diagnosis or the diagnosis was wrong. She would have been dead by now had she really had pancreatic cancer. People just don't spontaneously cure themselves."

"But, Dr. Marsh," Sam objected, "I've already seen things that just can't be explained by modern medicine; sick people that shouldn't have gotten better, but they did. How can we explain that?"

"Experience," he said simply. "You explain it through experience. No offense, but you simply don't have the experience to know when someone should get better or not. You see what you want to see. You haven't taken care of enough patients yet to realize that they do not find cure without us. Show me a patient who thinks they were cured through holistic or alternative means and I'll show you a patient that was either misdiagnosed or is crazy. People can't think away illness. If they could, there wouldn't be doctors."

"What about that man on the news last week?" asked one of the medical students. "He was waiting to board a plane at the airport when he developed chest pain and arrested. The woman standing in line behind him was a CCU nurse and resuscitated him. When he got out of the cardiac cath lab hours later, he learned that the plane he was going to board had crashed and that nobody survived, including the nurse that had saved his life. What message would you have us take from this?"

"That no good deed ever goes unpunished?" Ben suggested with a straight face. He let the shock register in the faces of his young colleagues for several moments before bursting into a laugh and continuing. "I'm joking, really," he said. "That's a great story, but I don't see any miracles in it. People have heart attacks every day and there is nothing the least bit surprising that a CCU nurse would know how to resuscitate him. There certainly isn't anything miraculous about a plane crashing. The fact that he wasn't on it was just luck.

"Dr. Marsh," began another resident, "when I was doing surgery in medical school, we had a patient about to have a lung resection for cancer. Before undergoing anesthesia, she insisted on having a central line placed. She didn't really need one, but rather than argue with her, the anesthesiologist put one in. A chest x-ray was done to confirm proper placement of the line, which it did, but it didn't show any traces of a tumor. An x-ray just weeks before showed a huge mass. That seems pretty miraculous to me. I mean, what are the odds of that happening?"

"Exactly the right question," Ben exclaimed, slapping the table with his hand, "what are the odds? It is simply a matter of statistics. A certain percentage of x-rays and even biopsies are read wrong. Clearly, this lady didn't have cancer, as cancer just doesn't disappear in a matter of weeks, even with treatment. But a certain percentage of lung infections or inflammation can look like cancer and those can disappear spontaneously. The miracle that you want to see is simply a manifestation of a poor understanding of statistics.

"It seems to me that the only criteria required for the proclamation of a miracle is that it's a rare event. Using that standard, if I come down here in the morning and find that the coffee is hot, I've just encountered a miracle. It's a religious experience if the coffee is actually good. The odds of winning the lottery are over three million to one. The odds of being struck by lightning are over a half-million to one. Does that make them miracles? Of course not, but yet we want to invoke metaphysics and guardian angles whenever a chest x-ray clears, something that's not all that uncommon."

Miracles; few topics can drive faculty physicians to greater angst.

Perhaps it's ego. It can be a powerful thing, sheltering our lives within a cocoon spun from self-import. Those of physicians though tend to be larger than most. There is a collective ego in medicine where the sum is so much greater than its many parts. It is an ego that thrives and grows ever stronger with the passage of time until it is left for a new generation to nourish with even greater advances in the science of cure.

With the stroke of a pen, antibiotics can be unleashed against organisms that once decimated civilizations, with a scalpel's edge mistakes of nature can be fixed, and through the thinnest of catheters, the spark of life can be restored to silent hearts. No wonder some physicians come to see themselves as invincible. Medicine is filled with apparent failure and unexpected success. The ego protects from both.

As difficult as failure can be to accept in medicine, it is unexpected success that many physicians struggle with the most. Despite the best that a teaching hospital has to offer, patients still die. It is a part of practicing medicine. The terminal cancer patient that lives, the paraplegic that somehow manages to walk, and the hopeless diagnosis that finds unlikely hope—events that evoke talk of miracles—however, can wage the fiercest battles with the ego of medicine. The possibility that their patients can get better without them is strangely threatening for many physicians. The physician speaks of placebo effects, observational bias, and errors of measurement to help explain the unexplainable. The alternative would be to believe in miracles. Clearly, Ben Marsh wasn't ready for such alternatives.

The conversation at the next table fascinated me. As I sat listening, the tradition of medicine was fulfilled—the philosophy of yesterday was offered to the keepers of today. No doubt, Ben taught as he had been taught and I wondered if his students would one day carry his philosophy of miracles into tomorrow. Looking at those young faces though, I wasn't so sure. They were thoughtful faces that seemed conflicted with doubt and uncertainty. The uncertainty thrilled me. Perhaps they were not yet ready to dismiss the possibility that miracles might touch their work. It is in being open to the possibility, no matter how slight it might seem, that miracles become possible.

The irony of my colleagues' discussion was not lost on me. While I always hadn't recognized it, my journey had been visited by miracles quite often through the practice of medicine. In fact, I had just shared that very morning with a miracle.

The medicine consult team was asked to see a young lady on the surgical service with elevated blood pressure. I thoroughly enjoyed the months that I was the attending physician for the medicine consult team. It was an opportunity to work closely with senior medical residents and to encounter clinical problems that we often did not encounter on the internal medicine service. Such was the case with Heather Scooter.

The weather had been as close to perfection as was possible for southern Ohio and it seemed more like summer that Sunday afternoon than early fall. The Scooter family wasn't going to waste a moment of it. While Heather's brother played football with friends in the backyard, her mother reveled in the garden. It was the finest in the neighborhood. Heather's dad was quite the landscaper and after a quick trip to the store for supplies, he planned to lose himself in mulch and pruning. As for Heather, she couldn't pass up what might be the last warm day of the year. With beach towel in hand, she set out to soak up some of the wonderful sunshine.

Dale Scooter had to give the SUV more gas than usual as he backed out of the sloping driveway. Typically, he had to press on the brakes to keep from going too fast. He didn't give it much thought until he reached the street and looked at the pile of trash in the middle of the driveway that he had obviously backed over. He shook his head slowly as scraps of cardboard and plastic flapped in the breeze, but he was determined that someone's negligence wasn't going to ruin the wonderful mood that he was in.

Something about that cardboard, however, made Dale take a second look. It almost looked like a foot and the piece of torn plastic looked amazingly like an arm and hand flailing in the air. He had seen those bright green and orange stripes before as well. It was the beach towel that his daughter always used when she would lay out in the sun. The recognition consumed every fiber of his body in the flames of panic and transformed his day, his entire life, in fact, instantly. He had run his daughter over with the car.

Heather's medical chart chronicled her journal from that driveway through her transport by medical helicopter, evaluation in the emergency department, and admission to the trauma service of the Teaching Hospital. The documentation was exquisite; every examination finding, procedure performed, and laboratory result was recorded. One page of the thick medical record caught my attention like none other ever had. It reached from the world of science and logic and touched a part of my heart that knew nothing of such things.

Trauma surgeons, while not always known for their skill at writing legible and informative chart notes, were great at drawing. On diagrams illustrating the front and back of the human body, every injury found during the admission examination was depicted in painstaking detail. I could only stare in surprise at the representation of Heather's injuries. Stretching from her left shoulder diagonally across her chest was an eight-inch-wide tread mark. Even the intricate pattern of the tire's tread was captured as if it had been left in moist sand.

I turned quickly to the surgery section of the chart to read about her outcome in the operating room, but found nothing there. I leafed through the nursing notes to determine how much blood she had required, but she hadn't received blood. The abnormalities I expected to find in her laboratory studies were not to be found. As impossible as it seemed, Heather's only injury was a fractured clavicle and bruised lungs. Was it luck, or something more?

Was it luck or perhaps a simple matter of statistics the morning Dawn Satchwell found herself in the hospital? As my ward team streamed into her room, she looked at the dawn sky through her bedside window with misgiving. She looked at us with surprise. It wasn't as she had intended. She was supposed to be dead.

Dawn's son, her only child, wanted to join the military for as long as she could remember. Her husband didn't want him to go. Her parents predicted disaster if he went. Her sister and brother were dumbfounded when shortly after his high-school graduation, Dawn supported his enlistment in the marines. She knew that he wouldn't have gone had she said no, but it was his dream.

With every newspaper that was delivered to the door, Dawn felt anxious. With every news broadcast, she trembled. She was uncommonly close to her son and feared for the worst. She feared for that which she could have prevented. When Dawn opened her front door to find two men in military uniforms standing on her porch, her fear became reality. A truck that her son was riding in had been destroyed in an explosion and there were no survivors.

The note that she left for her family told of an inability to face life without her son and that life with guilt was not worth living. She didn't consider herself a courageous person—that had been her son—so gently drifting off to sleep behind the wheel of her running car in the locked garage seemed the perfect solution. But the car wouldn't start. She never had trouble with the car before; in fact, it had just been serviced the week before. When she needed it the most, it failed her. Even her husband's handgun failed her. She knew it was loaded but for some reason she was unable to pull the trigger.

When a desperate husband found his wife, she was sitting unconscious in the front seat of her car. The interior lights did not turn on when he opened the door. Neither did the chimes sound, indicating that the keys were in the ignition. Apparently, the battery was dead.

His pistol lay in the passenger seat next to his wife and he breathed a sigh of relief when he realized it hadn't been fired. The safety was still on. Her lips and chin were streaked with a red material and large blotches stained the front of her blouse. It was sticky and had a sweet odor. An empty container of antifreeze lay on the floor at her feet.

Caring for suicide attempts was not unusual at the Teaching Hospital, but never before had I encountered someone that seemed so desperate to die. Never before had I encountered fate that seemed so destined to prevent it. The ethylene glycol in antifreeze is an effective killer and Dawn had consumed more than enough to do the job. But in the kitchen not far from her note was an empty bottle of vodka. Maybe it helped her find the courage to act upon her guilt, but it also saved her life. Ethanol is the antidote for antifreeze poisoning.

Dawn was very much alive that morning my team of residents and students gathered around her bed. She was also very deaf and we could not explain why. When all of her examinations and tests were found to be normal, the consulting psychiatrist hypothesized conversion hysteria as the cause. Her loss of hearing was simply a reflection of the profound guilt she felt in her son's death, and perhaps the guilt that she felt in still being alive.

Three days after her world was quieted, Dawn's hearing returned. It happened as suddenly and as mysteriously as it had left. While most would find elation at such a happening, Dawn seemed rather matter-of-fact about the whole thing, perhaps even a little wistful, and I attributed it to her depression. When I mentioned it to Dawn, she assured me she wasn't depressed, at least not any more. She found the days that she spent in silence strangely fulfilling and felt calm seldom experienced during her life. Quiet had always been unsettling to Dawn. She found comfort in noise and always drove to work with the radio on or passed the hours at home, never far from a television. Somehow, it was always preferable to being left alone with her thoughts.

The silence imposed through illness though reminded her a little of the battles she had fought with her parents over spinach when she was a child—once she finally tried it, she rather liked it. Alone with her thoughts, perhaps for the first time, she discovered just how much noise they too could make. As the hours passed, her thoughts came less often; between those thoughts was incredible tranquility and insight. While she didn't fully understand it, she felt a connection with everything that has ever been and everything that will ever be and knew beyond any doubt that her life was unfolding as it should. So too had her son's life and she spoke of finding great contentment in the realization that it was not yet his time and that he still had work to do.

If the suicide attempt wasn't enough to earn Dawn admission to the psychiatric unit, the peace and understanding she described through her deafness made it the highest of priorities. It was the day she was transferred to psychiatry that word reached Dawn's family from he military. The vehicle in which her son had been riding in was not the one that had been destroyed. While injured and in a military hospital, he was expected to live.

Where the psychiatrist found coincidence, luck, and the disordered thoughts of mental illness, I was sure I could see miracles. Perhaps it was in a car that wouldn't start, a gun that wouldn't fire, or a poison rendered harmless. Perhaps it was in a military vehicle not ridden in. Perhaps the incomprehensible is the universe's miraculous way to guide us to a silent place where there is understanding.

There comes a time in a physician's journey when statistical distribution just can't explain the unexpected cure, when luck seems an inadequate reason for averted tragedy, and coincidence falls far short of explaining the unexplainable. There comes a time, however brief it might be, when something greater than their touch seems to ease a pain or calm a life. In that moment, they can witness miracles. Some, if they are open to the possibility, can even participate in them. Such was the case when Daniel Stein shared his path with me.

He was a quiet and unassuming man when we first met in my office. Having recently moved to the area, he was looking for a new physician. He had retired from the military several years earlier and had recently embarked on a new career as a teacher. He seemed to like teaching, but I suspected it was a life that was taking some getting used to.

Daniel was an easy person to talk to but there was never much depth in what he shared about himself. He was a rather healthy middle-aged man taking medication for high blood pressure and elevated cholesterol. He had some nagging stiffness and joint pain from injuries that he sustained when he was in the service, but he viewed them as nothing more than nuisances.

While it would be many months until I would learn that those injuries were caused by an airplane crash, it would take years for the whole story to unfold—a story I had been certain was hidden beneath his calm surface from the moment I met Daniel. He wasn't even supposed to be on the plane; in fact, it took much finagling for him to arrange to be onboard. He wanted on that flight so much that he gladly tolerated spending the night on a cramped and uncomfortable supply transport just to meet up with it.

Open training slots were rare and always inconvenient in the military, but it was worth a fair amount of pain in order to gain experience on new equipment that most assuredly led to career advancement.

The flight hadn't made it to its halfway point when Daniel began to have doubts about his choice of training assignments. They were flying into a large weather system and the turbulence was enough to unnerve even the veterans among the crew. As they descended toward their destination, there was no longer any doubt; it had been a huge mistake. Sitting in the cockpit's jump seat behind the pilots, Daniel could see nothing but white through the windows. The fierce winter storm buffeted the aircraft about like a toy and had he not been so frightened, he most certainly would have become sick. If the visibility ever improved, it was only moments before the plane hit the ground hundreds of feet short of the runway.

Three men died that night amidst flames and snow. Daniel and the pilots made it out with relatively minor injuries compared to those that rode in back, but I suspected the deepest wounds that would take the longest to heal were ones that could not be seen. What Daniel didn't tell me was that he was responsible for getting the pilots to safety before the plan erupted in flames. It was a detail shared by

Daniel's wife and I wondered what other mysteries might be found behind those quiet eyes.

During one of his visits to the office, Daniel and I were discussing a newspaper article about a local lady that had won the lottery for the third time and how some people just seemed to have good luck and others bad. I asked him if his selection of the doomed training flight ever made him think of himself as unlucky.

"I'm not sure it was bad luck," he replied. "At times I think it was a miracle."

Over the years, Daniel and his wife blended into the obscurity of my practice, seldom coming to the office for anything other than routine checks of his blood pressure and cholesterol. So I found it unusual one weekend morning in late autumn when Daniel called me at home. I had just seen him in the office a week or two earlier, and as usual, he was doing great.

"I'm really embarrassed to bother you about this," he started, "but I've had the strangest numbness in my toes the past couple of days. I noticed it in my left foot yesterday morning when I woke up. I thought I had just slept wrong and that it was asleep. But today I've got the same thing in both feet."

He laughed when I told him he was doing me a huge favor by calling, that I really didn't like French toast anyway and that the coffee was cold. Although I hadn't a clue as to the cause of the numbness, his recent exam and normal blood work reassured me and I suggested that we watch things for a day or two. By the next morning, however, Daniel reported that both feet were now entirely numb.

"You had a flu shot when you were in the office, didn't you?" I asked.

"Yes, but what does that have to do with anything?" he replied.

"I don't have the flu."

"Probably nothing," I said, "but I would like to see you in the emergency room."

"I'm not going to the hospital for numb feet," he gasped in disbelief. "I probably just pinched a nerve somewhere."

I reluctantly agreed to another day of observation, but when he described a tingling sensation across both shins, I was filled with profound worry. Despite my insistence, he remained stubborn in his refusal to go the hospital.

"Look, Mr. Stein," I said in a firm voice, "you need to trust me on this one."

"Wow," he replied in surprise, "you haven't called me Mr. Stein in years. Okay, I'll go to the hospital, but under protest."

By the following morning, Daniel could not feel anything below his knees and needed help walking to the chair in his room.

"It's called Guillain Barre," I told a mystified-appearing Daniel that night in his hospital room. "It's a rare, but not unheard of, complication from the influenza vaccine. Everyone's case is a little different so it's hard to tell you just what to expect, but the paralysis is likely to get worse. It tends to move up the body, and in some goes on to affect the respiratory system. If that would happen, you would need to be placed on a ventilator—a machine that would breathe for you—until you get better.

"The good news is that most people do get better. The neurologists are going to be giving you medication that increases that likelihood. The bad news is that it is going to take a long time to get better. Once the paralysis resolves, you need to learn how to use everything again. Most need to spend time in a rehabilitation center."

Daniel asked no questions and showed little emotion. There was fear, however, in those quiet eyes. It was subtle and I would have missed it had he not offered an occasional glimpse into the mysteries of his life over the years.

"Whatever the days ahead might bring, Daniel," I added with a squeeze of his hand, "we will walk them together. You will not be alone."

Daniel faced the relentless progression of loss with stoicism. It was like watching a man fall off a high cliff in slow motion and knowing that he knew he would eventually hit the ground. On the third hospital day, with paralysis having progressed to the waist, Daniel was moved to the Intensive Care Unit. On the fourth day, I sat next to his bed—my science powerless to help—as a ventilator was wheeled into the room. Through it, he maintained a frightened silence.

Daniel spent a week on the ventilator before his ravaged nervous system began to heal. When healthy enough to withstand the rigors of therapy, Daniel was transferred to the finest rehabilitation center in the region. There he started to regain all that he had taken for granted in his life.

It would be close to four months before Daniel was once again sitting in my office. With persistence and many more weeks of outpatient therapy, he was finally able to discard the cane that had steadied his walk for much of his journey. The numbness and tingling in the tips of his toes, however, would never go away. His doctors called it peripheral neuropathy. He called it a precious reminder of the gift of today.

Routine quickly returned to our lives and it wouldn't be long until our office visits were once again focused on blood pressure measurements and cholesterol levels. The Daniel that came to those visits, however, was subtly different than the man I had known before. He seemed happier and so much more at peace since his illness. I commented on it one day when he was getting ready to leave the office.

"Strange that you would say that," he observed. "My wife said the same thing just the other night. I don't think I feel happier; life has been pretty good to me. It's just that things make more sense to me these days. I understand why I am here and where I am going even though I cannot put it into words.

"I need to tell you something that I haven't told anyone before. I was afraid people would think I was crazy. When I was in the plane crash, I had help getting out. It was pitch black in that cockpit and I wasn't familiar with where anything was located. I couldn't have saved myself let alone those pilots. The strangest thing happened. A light seemed to form right in front of me. It was a brilliant white light, but even though we were in darkness, it didn't hurt my eyes. I had just experienced the most terrifying event of my life but that light made me feel unusually calm. The light moved up and toward the center of the cockpit and illuminated an emergency hatch in the ceiling. I never would have known it was there. It was the hatch that I took the pilots through.

"Was the light that I saw in that plane from the fire? It's what I've always tried to convince myself of, even though the plane did not explode until we made it out. But now I know differently because I've seen that light again."

"Where?" I asked. "When?"

"In the hospital after I got sick," he said. "I was terrified. I think I was more frightened than I was when I was on that plane. It was when I was in the Intensive Care Unit when they brought the breathing machine in my room. That same light was next to my bed. It spoke to me and seemed to know exactly what was going to happen to me. It assured me that I would be alright and promised that it would never be far away and I would never be alone.

"Just like on that plane, my fear disappeared instantly. I knew that everything would turn out fine and all I needed to do was let go and let it happen. Then the light changed. It became softer and took on the shape of a person. When it disappeared, you were standing in its place. I didn't have a moment of fear after that moment. In its place was left nothing but stillness. I could actually feel myself healing. You were responsible for that. You were the light."

"You give me more credit than I deserve, Daniel," I said softly and feeling more than a little self-conscious. "I didn't do anything; there wasn't anything I could do. I just happened to be there."

"There was no happenstance about it. You chose to be there. Don't you think it strange that with all the specialists, fancy tests, and expensive medication that it would be your presence and words I remember most, which brought me the greatest comfort? Well, I don't; not any more. I think technology has made us smug and we have lost sight of what's important in healthcare. How is it that you know just what to give in order to help someone? You certainly didn't learn it from a book. It's miraculous really."

"I've been thinking a lot about miracles recently. Maybe people are the miracles. On that airplane, I was the miracle just as you were the miracle in my hospital room."

The sound of a metal tray crashing to the floor startled me and brought my attention back to the hospital coffee shop and the discussion of miracles at the next table.

"Maybe you're right, Dr. Marsh," I heard Sam say. "Maybe we do only see what we want to find, but don't you think the opposite it true as well; that we will never see what we really don't want to find?

Are there not times in medicine when we accomplish things that we shouldn't be able to do, when the outcome of our patients surpass our ability to understand, and when we find ourselves in awe? Perhaps these are the miracles. If we never consider the possibility that there is more than that which we know about and are comfortable with, we may never experience that awe. What a shame it would be to go through medicine without that."

Silence fell over the crowded table as mystified-looking faces contemplated the unknown. Even Ben Marsh was silent, a rather miraculous event in and of itself. It was the silence from which miracles seem possible and there was no doubt in my mind that these young physicians would look for something that their teachers could not find. I was swept with an almost overwhelming sense of hope that morning because I knew they would find what they looked for.

CHAPTER 11

Life is a Lottery

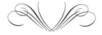

The spirit is life. The mind is the builder. This physical is the result.

EDGAR CAYCE

Beware what you set your heart upon. For it shall surely be yours.

RALPH WALDO EMERSON

I often find my thoughts visiting that ancient Buddhist proverb—
when the student is ready the teacher will appear. It wasn't until
I wandered the rises and falls of Demazie Hollow that I started to
appreciate the profound wisdom of those words. I met many of my
teachers here—some I had first encountered only recently while
others have waited countless years for just the right moment for when
their lessons might be understood.

Betts Unger was one of those teachers. Long before I had an
inkling of a path to take upon my journey, she knew the direction
my life would eventually be pulled. Even before I was prepared to
understand, she introduced me to the mysteries of energy, healing,
and manifesting—ingredients of the extraordinary—so that I might
be ready for that which awaited me.

Seldom would I look upon the immense red oak that towered over the clearing in Demazie Hollow that I would not see Betts waiting for me. It was not unlike the oak that stood at the edge of the marsh where Betts taught me about birds and about life. There was a fallen log beneath its canopy upon which we sat and peered into the world that surrounded us. Despite the confusion of woven grasses and tangled vines, the view through our binoculars always seemed uncommonly clear.

I had thought that my relationship with Betts was all about birds, but now as I leaf through brittle and yellowing pages of a notebook written in the hand of a boy some forty years ago, I know it was much more. It was about abundance—abundance that was ours for the seeking on every trip—and how to attract it into our lives. Betts was a master teacher of life. Through her, I developed a reverence for nature and began to appreciate the healing energy from which it flows. It shouldn't have come as a surprise to me that I would hear her lessons so clearly in the quiet of the hollow. It was as if she knew where my journey would lead and waited along the trail for me to catch up. Just as Betts and I discovered birds on every trail, it can be same with life; we find what we look for.

The abundance that Betts taught me to see was everywhere in Damazie Hollow, but so too was the apparent scarcity that plagued those that lived among the hills and valleys nearby. It was a disparity that always troubled me and was never far from my thoughts when working in the free clinic or driving to or from the hollow. The people of the area—probably not much different than people anywhere—viewed their lot in life as either *Lucky or Unlucky.*

Delbert Crady was among the latter. The aging man lived on the ridge not far from me and while nobody really knew how old he was,

I was rather certain that he appeared much older than he actually was. Years spent in scarcity do that to the body. He was an irritable man and I remember his first visit to the clinic vividly.

"Life is a damn lottery," he grumbled as he sat down in a worn chair in the corner of the examination room, "and I lost."

His problem list was long and matched what I expected in a man who seemed to have far too little on which to live. His emphysema made it difficult to walk at times and even if he believed that his smoking made it worse, it was one of the few pleasures he claimed in life. His startling high blood pressure readings suggested that he didn't take the medications we had arranged for the drug company to provide free of charge. We stopped doing finger-sticks to measure his blood sugar, as there was little hope he would follow a diet or take his pills. He seemed immune from the benefits of nature that surrounded his life on the ridge.

"Let me tell you about nature," he said one day in response to my probing about the good fortune he had to live in such a beautiful place. "I'd much rather have a room in the city than be stuck out in the middle of nowhere. Nothing is easy out there. You can't eat trees or pay bills with beauty. And about that beauty; I've been stuck out there for years and have yet to see it.

"I thought I could make a little money by digging ginseng last year. So I get bit by a copperhead—twice. Every morning I can't sleep because of the racket those blackbirds make. The more of them I shoot, the more that takes their place and the louder they get. Oh, and about those beautiful trees in the spring? The pollen is so bad I can't breathe for months. I'd cut them all down but there're just too many of them. They grow like weeds out there. Give me a room in the city any day."

I was bewildered by his tirade but would come to learn it was vintage Delbert Crady. Seldom had I met an unhappier man and I was at a loss to know how I might help him. He stopped coming to the clinic and upon investigating why, I learned that his battle with nature had raged on and had gone very badly for him.

Every year in early spring, the hills of Appalachia are blessed with a delicacy known only to a few. Apparently, the allure of morel mushrooms sautéed in butter was greater than his distaste for the woods that he had to traverse to harvest them. Perhaps it was bait for a well-laid trap, but it was the largest mushroom he had ever seen. As he bent to pluck it from the forest floor, his foot slipped on a moist rock, causing him to fall hard to the ground. He knew his leg was broken; the snap was as loud as a gunshot. It took the better part of the day for him to crawl out from the woods.

It was a bad fracture and required surgery. Every several days, visiting nurses would stop by his home to change his dressings and attend to his needs, but Delbert was unaccustomed to being attended to. It didn't take long for him to chase away all who came to help. But it was help that he desperately needed and without it he did not do well. By the time he returned to the hospital, his infected wound was beyond the reach of antibiotics and he lost his leg. Delbert lived out the rest of his life in a home barely large enough for his wheelchair. Most would have missed walks in the woods or strolls along the road, but from his wheelchair, Delbert received life as he expected it would come.

Not far away on the very same ridge, Mabel Satchwell tended her gardens. Like Delbert, she had little money, and her small home was in need of repair and the modern conveniences that those in the city would take for granted. She had lived in the country all of her life, but she saw something different than Delbert when she looked out across the fields and woods. She too often thought of life as a lottery, but it was one she had clearly won.

If I struggled to remember a time when I saw Delbert Crady with a smile, there was never a time when I would see Mabel without one. She too came to the clinic and had her share of problems. Arthritis had stiffened her legs and twisted her hands but she managed to find something to smile about even in that. While even simple tasks took longer than they once did, it only meant she could spend longer in her garden.

Her gardens were spectacular. No matter how fickle the season—with earth-cracking heat in the driest of summers to soil sodden with endless spring rains—Mabel's gardens were always lush and vibrant. For a handful of seeds and a little work that never seemed much like work, the bounty seemed endless. While she didn't understand the universal laws that might explain abundance, she lived with it daily and was grateful for it.

Mabel's garden was never depleted or her pantry ever empty when visitors would stop. As soon as a tomato would be picked, a new one would seem to grow in its place. There was always one more jar of preserves that she didn't remember putting up. The corn was always sweeter when it was shared with her neighbors.

"You can never run out," she scoffed one day when I suggested that perhaps she should keep more for herself. Clearly, I had much to learn about abundance. Mabel received life as she expected it would come.

There was no better place to learn about abundance than Demazie Hollow. Whatever my spirit needed the most—an uncommon bird, the simplicity of a wildflower, or tranquil sanctuary—it never failed to appear there and I came to realize that abundance, or scarcity, was what we attract in life. When diagnoses are slow to come at the hospital or answers elude problems in the office, solutions are never far away. The energy found in our special places is powerful and for those that know how to use it, there is no limit to the wonders they can attract into their lives. Mabel was one such person but there have been many other teachers. Often they appear for only brief moments, but their lessons can be so startling that you know the way you look at life will never be quite the same. A few such moments on a summer afternoon will be with me forever.

I groaned when I got out of my car and read the sign taped to the gasoline pump—*Pay At Pump Out of Order. Please pay inside when finished.* It had been a long day in the office and I was anxious to get home. I never went inside to pay for gasoline; I was always too busy for that. It was the only pump available so with a sigh of resignation and an indignant glance toward the cashier, I set about filling the car with fuel.

I'm not sure that I ever encountered a slower gasoline pump and my irritation built with every update of the pump's display. I looked at my watch incredulously—thirty seconds to pump a gallon—it would take ten minutes to fill up the car. I cleaned the windshield and checked the tires. I even checked the oil, something I seldom did any more. Somewhere during the waiting and the chores, I realized how hot it was.

It was the first hot spell of summer. Unusual for the temperature to rise above ninety in early June, the temperature had done so for the third straight day. Already breaking records, I wondered what the hot part of summer would bring. As I walked across the parking lot to pay for the gasoline, I noticed that the heat radiating from the asphalt penetrated the soles of my shoes and warmed my feet.

Before I could make it to the store's door, an old and rusted red pickup truck lurched to a stop at the curb, a thick black cloud of exhaust pouring from the tailpipe, which hung suspended by a piece of twisted clothes hanger. The dented driver's side door creaked open and slammed shut, and I watched with irritation as a man raced into the store ahead of me. Sure enough, even though he hadn't pumped any gasoline or made a selection from the store's shelves, he stood in front of me in line for the cashier.

He was an older man, although like most I encountered in the hills of the country, I suspected his coarse features and weathered hands made him appear older than he actually was. He stood with a stoop and shifted his weight impatiently from one leg to the other. He looked as rushed as I felt. He also looked out of place—his long-sleeved flannel shirt and worn jeans seemingly more appropriate for a cool autumn day. His thinning gray hair hung far below his collar, but I doubted it was a style of his choice.

As we waited, the stranger's hands fidgeted nervously in his pockets that were obviously filled with coins. When it was finally his turn and he stepped to the counter, the young man at the cash register recognized him with a smile. "George," he said, "it's been a long time. How are you doing in this heat?"

The old man, clearly embarrassed by the attention, mumbled a response that I strained to hear.

"I only come when I really need something," he said almost apologetically. "I can take the heat but the wife's got it bad. It's hard for her to breathe since our air conditioner broke. None of her medicines seem to help."

My irritation at this old man melted away to sympathy as I

watched him pull a clenched fist from his pocket and plunk a couple of crumpled dollar bills and a pile of coins upon the counter. From the other pocket he withdrew still more coins and added them to the pile.

Pointing to the glass display case, he asked, "Do I have enough for one of those?"

As the ever-growing line watched and waited, the cashier slowly counted the man's money and pushed a few coins back toward him. "You have seventeen cents too much, George," he said. As the old man returned the coins to the safety of his pocket, I couldn't help but believe it was all the money he had left to his name. I was shocked when I saw the cashier reach for the instant lottery tickets, realizing for the first time what the old man had come to buy.

I heard a voice from deep within me. It was a voice I thought I had banned from my life long ago, but there it was—a voice of judgment and scorn.

As the cashier tore a lottery ticket from the roll in the display case, the old man looked down at his feet with a mixture of embarrassment and perhaps shame. "Could I have the next one instead?" he asked. If the cashier was annoyed, he didn't show it. Instead, he tore the next ticket from the roll and handed it to the man who had intruded so deeply into my life.

Without a moment's pause the old man anxiously scratched away at the card, then without even looking at it, handed it back to the cashier. With a smile and a twinkle in his eye, the cashier called his manager from the office. The now impressively long line stood in shocked silence as the manager counted out five hundred dollars to the old man.

With a humble thank you and trembling hands, the man picked up the bills and rushed from the store.

LIFE IS A LOTTERY

"He was in a few months ago and won a hundred dollars on the fifty-cent game," the cashier told us as we watched that old red truck disappear down the road in a cloud of smoke.

It didn't seem all that hot when I left the store a few minutes later. Strange, but I didn't feel rushed either. The treadmill upon which my life had been running for far too long slowed that afternoon, just enough to meet a special teacher.

"When the student is ready," the words ran through my thoughts, "the teacher will appear." And there he went, on his way to buy his wife an air conditioner.

CHAPTER 12

It was Only a Moment Ago

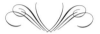

*The past is but the beginning of a beginning, and all that
is and has been is but the twilight of the dawn.*

H.G. WELLS

*Most men lead lives of quiet desperation and go
to the grave with the song still in them.*

HENRY DAVID THOREAU

I wish I had paid closer attention while taking physics in college
because then I might be better able to explain some of the unexplainable that occurs with surprising frequency in medicine. I wish I
had filled my undergraduate years with literature as the wisdom from
those who came before us might have brought clarity to the confusion
of a physician's day. I wish I would have learned more about philosophy
and theology during those years of study, for then I might have better
seen the soul behind the patient. Pre-medicine curriculum, however,
is more about memorization of facts and test scores that will garner
admission to medical school than it is about preparing one for a life
of healing. That task had to fall to my greatest teachers: my patients.

Few things have introduced greater contradiction along my journey than time. Often, it has been a bitter enemy; determined to deprive hectic days a sense of accomplishment. Other times it has shown the compassion of a close friend in providing the opportunity to touch the soul hiding behind the frightened eyes of a diagnosis. Sometimes it passes painfully slow, but more often than not, it slips unnoticed into tomorrow.

Of the countless problems my patients have brought to my office over the years—disease and despair, pain and sorrow, and the loss of youth—time has been their greatest threat to health and happiness. It has also become one of my most important tools of healing.

Craig Jasper stopped by the office one day hoping to be seen for a sore knee. He wasn't a patient and he didn't have an appointment, but his kind face touched the heart of my assistant and she promised to work him for a few minutes just before we left for lunch. After all, it was only for a sore knee.

Indeed, Mr. Jasper had a kind face but it was clouded with pain. His knee just started to hurt the day or so before. He didn't recall any injuries and while he worked hard every day, he hadn't done anything out of the ordinary. What he thought most strange was that he felt better when he was using it. When he would stop to rest, the constant dull ache would set in again. It was worse at night and the pain was keeping him from sleeping. He wondered if it might be arthritis. His mother had arthritis and it usually bothered her when the seasons changed. He thought he remembered his knee bothering him around the same time the year before.

Despite his obvious discomfort—he walked to the exam room with a limp—I couldn't find anything wrong with his knee. In fact, he had the best-looking knees I had seen all day, but then again, at thirty-seven, he was the first person under the age of sixty I had seen all day. There was no tenderness, inflammation, and not the slightest evidence of discomfort to my manipulations. He seemed reassured by my belief that he most likely had an overuse injury and would get better with rest and perhaps some anti-inflammatory medications.

As he turned to leave, I asked him if he was heading back to work or if he had the rest of the day off. It was one of those questions we ask simply to fill time and one that I wasn't particularly interested in the answer. I certainly wasn't prepared for it.

"No," he said with resignation in his voice, "I need to run out to the cemetery. I've been putting it off. It's just a hard trip to make."

"Parents?" I asked.

"No, my son," he said quietly. "He was three when he died; two years ago today as a matter of fact."

I looked up from his chart that I had been writing in with a start. I thought I must have heard him wrong, but the tear in his eye told me I had not. I motioned to the chair that he had been sitting in and he sat back down, albeit reluctantly. I was mortified that I could miss something so obvious. I had thought the problem was his knee, but it wasn't. It was time.

Craig was at work when the telephone call came. His home had caught on fire. His girlfriend had made it out but his little boy hadn't. The paramedics took him to the hospital and while they did everything they could to save his son, it wasn't enough.

It was the day of the funeral when the social worker came. Craig struggled to explain what he himself couldn't understand to his eldest son who stood by his side as sad-looking friends slowly made their way to their cars. The second grader was safely at school when the fire started, but he would not be spared its aftermath that would forever change his life. It had already been decided by those who knew best. Craig was obviously a bad father and could not be trusted with the precious life of another child. Craig never learned where the county social workers placed his child and he was not permitted visitation. It was for the child's best, he was assured. He never saw his son again.

If I had struggled to find a solution for the pain in Craig's knee, I could make no sense of the pain that filled his life. All I could do was sit in subdued silence and listen. There would be no lunch that day.

Maxwell Woodson was sitting in the waiting room when Craig left. He too had an illness of time. I had never met a more miserable person. On each visit, the sixty-year-old banker would tell me how many more months he had until retirement. While the thought of not having to go to work each day would bring a smile to most faces, the closer he got to retirement the unhappier he seemed. In the preceding months, he had been treated for peptic ulcer disease, worsening hypertension, headaches, back pain, and palpitations.

"I don't get it," I said to him one day, "don't you want to retire?"

"I can't wait," he responded. "I only have eighteen-months left."

"Then why do you seem so stressed?" I pressed. "You are wound tighter than anyone I've seen. When was your last vacation?"

"It's been years," he said. "Maybe I am a little tired, but there will be plenty of time to take it easy in eighteen months. It's going to be great. We are going to travel and spend time with the grandkids. I've always wanted to do woodworking, so I'm going to make a shop in the garage. I even have a list of books I'm going to read. Things will be better soon."

"Things will better soon," I repeated, "but what of today? What if today was all that you had?"

I have grown fascinated with time. Thousands of patients have come and gone along my journey. Some I have known for only brief moments while others have lingered throughout much of my discovery of healing. Some have died as old friends after lives fulfilled with rich understanding and captured dreams, while others passed far too young, before really knowing what their dreams were. Be it measured in decades or years, our time here in this place is brief.

The box turtle that steps softly across the floor of Demazie Hollow—with a life that spans more than a century—will live longer than most of my patients. The giant red oak that stands watch over that sacred place was but a sapling when settlers came from the east. The ammonite fossil that sits on my desk speaks with a voice some 180 million years old. In the perspective of the universe we come, live, and go all in the blink of an eye.

There is a remarkable paradox in the brevity of now—it will last forever. There has never been a time that hasn't been now and there will never be a time when it is not now. It's an incredible gift for those whose time is short. Life happens now, but it can be lost in yesterday or misspent waiting for tomorrow. Happiness is found in the present moment.

Craig Jasper and Maxwell Woodson suffered the same disease. They lived their lives in a place other than now—where happiness can never be found. The pain and sadness that Craig found in the past made it impossible to find what life offers in the present moment. There is no guarantee of tomorrow. Life can change in the blink of an eye. It was a difficult reality for Maxwell. Rather than experience the pleasures that life could bring today, he gambled it all on a day that may never come.

Just as my teachers taught me about the power found in the present moment, they helped me come to understand how to find it. There are some activities that by their very nature can only take place in the present moment. When we pause to appreciate beauty—a tree in bloom, the notes of a symphony, or a painting on a wall—our thoughts are pulled back from that which might await us, or from that which has already been, to the instant of now. It is where beauty is found. Moments spent in gratitude, no matter how fleeting, are spent in the present moment. When we give something of ourselves to others—a generous tip at a restaurant, a moment to listen, or helping a neighbor with a chore—it happens now, not yesterday or tomorrow. When we find the stillness within us so that we can hear the silence, we have found the present moment. The longer we spend each day here, the more special it becomes.

That time has direction—from the age of the ammonite fossils, through the present moment, and on to the futures that we dream about—finds comfort in the rational mind, even if our briefest of appearances along that continuum is rather disconcerting. My teachers have told of another type of time and had I paid closer attention in those college physics classes, perhaps I would have been open to the possibility of non-linear time much earlier in my journey. I didn't understand much about Einstein's Theory of Relativity, quantum mechanics, or Heisenberg's Uncertainty Principle, but I was in good company. I still find it exhilarating that our greatest scientific minds are only now starting to understand the fundamental mysteries of the universe.

While I would gradually surrender my belief in coincidence and chance that was cultured through years of traditional education and training, it would be some time before I was ready to see the marvels of time that played out around me. That time might have currents and intelligence to its flow seemed more appropriate for the world of the spiritualist than that of the physician, but the synchronicity that I saw in medicine could not be denied. It was a healing energy and I felt it particularly strong when Heidi Goff visited my office one day.

I had seen Mrs. Goff several times before, but knew little of her past. The seventy-two-year-old lady had a thick German accent and I always thought that the hills of Appalachia was a strange place for her to have settled. She was a healthy woman and as it was on previous visits, we finished our business with plenty of time to sit and chat for a while—so I asked her about her past. Through the words that followed, she became one of my teachers.

While my memories of childhood are filled with family, vacations, and abundance, Heidi's were consumed by war and its aftermath. She grew up during the Second World War and spent much of that time in harm's way, although she grew oblivious to it. Her family lived aboard a supply boat that her father operated on the Rhine River. His job was to ferry supplies from ships anchored in deep water to destinations in shallow waters upriver. It was a horrible place for a family to be—aboard what was considered a military target.

When the war was at its peak, hardly a week would pass when they were not bombed. Sometimes it happened several times a day. They would hear the planes long before they saw them. They always seemed to fly up river, probably with any bombs that might have been left over from attacks on the big ships at anchor. In the beginning, the kids would all take cover beneath deck but as the attacks grew more common, they often watched from above. After all, where could you hide on a boat? The planes flew low enough that Heidi could see their propellers spin. She could see the bombs as they fell through the air.

It was not usual for the stories of my patients to touch me deeply, but with increasing regularity, they left me stunned and aware of the extraordinary moments that weave throughout our lives. I could only sit and look into the smiling eyes that as a child saw challenge that few adults will ever come to know.

"It must have been terrifying," I managed to say after many moments of silence.

"Not really," she said. "It might have been at first but mostly I was excited when the planes came."

"I beg your pardon?" I asked.

"It was wartime and food wasn't all that plentiful. When the planes came, I knew we would eat well that day. I guess hunger trumps fear, even in a little girl."

She laughed at the quizzical expression on my face and said, "It was the bombs. When they would hit the water and explode, dozens of dead fish would rise up to the surface. We were always ready with nets when the planes came. People would come from shore—in motor boats, rowboats, and some even by wading—desperate to try to get a fish. It was food. Those bombs were a gift from God."

Bombs as a gift from God; the mere possibility sent a chill up my spine. That grace could be found in the midst of such catastrophe profoundly moved me and I knew without a moment's doubt I was sharing in wisdom from a place where time is meaningless.

"It wasn't until after the war," Heidi continued, "that I discovered real hunger. There was no food. Most days we were fortunate to have some bread and maybe some scraps of meat to eat once a day. I remember stealing food once. I had never stolen anything in my life—and never have since—but I was just so hungry. Living with that guilt was worse than being hungry.

"When there wasn't enough food, my father always told us that he wasn't hungry, but I could see the hunger in his eyes as he watched us kids devour whatever was placed in front of us. I saw something else in those eyes. I always thought I knew what love was—telling family that you loved them was second nature in my family—but it wasn't until I saw those eyes that I really knew. There can be no greater depiction of love than wanting something more for others than you want for yourself, even if it is something that you might desperately need.

"I'm so very fortunate. Some people live their entire lives without ever knowing what true love is. I've gone through most of my life knowing. As horrible as that war was, I might never have experienced such purity of life had I not lived through those years. I try to remember that whenever times seem hard. It has been a blessing."

There were tears in my eyes as Heidi shared her story with me. I had encountered many teachers along my travels; most I would not recognize as such until long afterwards. Some, no doubt, still linger in the deep recesses of my memories waiting for that moment of silence when they might be remembered and their gifts recognized. There have been times, however, when my journey has taken a high road and I can see farther and clearer than usual. Perhaps I am simply starting to enjoy the trip and am more open to the wonders that can be found along the way. It is during these times there can be no doubt when special teachers come to us. I knew Heidi was one such teacher and that her lessons were as extraordinary as they were timeless. That great beauty can be made possible through the darkest of life's turns was exciting and strangely comforting.

As Heidi settled herself in the waiting room to await a ride home, I got ready to see my next patient. I had kept him waiting, but I didn't seem to care. My time with Heidi could not have been better spent. I smiled when I walked into the next exam room and saw Jeff Corse sitting there. The eighty-four-year-old man appeared as he always had—a broad grin across his weathered face and a baseball cap with military insignia pulled down over his eyes.

I had seen Jeff many times and each visit added to my understanding of the man who had intrigued me so over the years. Aside from the blue jeans, flannel work shirt, and even the ball cap, he always seemed to belong behind an executive desk in the city rather than the fields and hills of the country. Some fifteen years earlier, he had, in fact, retired from a corporate job in the city to return to the country. He had been raised on a farm and the pull of nature and open spaces grew too strong to resist. He always thought retirement would one day take him home again, but something fascinated him about this place and he found a new home many hundreds of miles from his roots.

Jeff was the first in his family ever to go to college. It was quite a feat for a farm boy and while he felt a little guilty about leaving the never-ending chores to his brothers, he followed the path that opportunity had provided. After college and a few years in the service, he got a job as an engineer with a large defense contractor. It wasn't long until he did his work from a leather chair.

"Jeff," I said, "this is an unexpected surprise. I hope everything is alright; we just saw you last month."

"I don't know why I'm here," he said, shaking his head. "I'm probably just wasting your time."

"Hold on now," I said softly, "it's me you're talking to. Even if we just sit and talk, it will be well worth it. Now why don't you tell me what it is I can do for you?"

"That's the problem," he said, relaxing a bit, "I don't know. Something just doesn't seem right. I don't think I'm sleeping well. I've never had problems sleeping before. I think I need sleeping pills. The past three nights I've had the strangest dreams; but I don't dream. This isn't me."

"If you're dreaming," I reasoned, "then you must be sleeping. What are the dreams about?"

"About war and children," he said, clearly frustrated. "It's probably because of that documentary I saw on television last week. It was about civilian casualties during war. They kept showing these pictures of children who were killed or horribly wounded. Every night I see faces of children that I hurt during the war. They ask me why, but I don't know why."

"You served, didn't you?" I asked. "What war was it?"

"The Second World War," he replied, "I was recruited right out of college; a twenty-one-year-old kid that didn't know a thing."

"That was a long time ago, Jeff," I observed.

"That's just it," he insisted. "It was only a moment ago. I remember everything like it happened yesterday—the name of the cook in the mess, the telephone number of the girl I met in town, the tune that my bunkmate whistled. It just happened."

"Where did you serve?" I asked. "What did you do?"

"In Europe toward the end of the war," he said with a hint of a smile. "I was in the Army Air Corps. They took a bunch of us college kids, made us first lieutenants, and taught us how to fly. Most of the guys I trained with shipped off to the South Pacific, but I had it pretty easy. Things were winding down by the time I made it to Europe. We took some antiaircraft fire, but I never did encounter an enemy fighter during my entire tour.

"It wasn't bad duty at all. It was like a nine-to-five job; there was always a hot meal waiting at the end of the day. It was quite beautiful actually. The scenery from my cockpit was simply spectacular, and at times, I felt guilty that I enjoyed the missions so much. I never did see war close up. I've always considered that a blessing—until now."

"Why is that?" I asked.

"Maybe because war shouldn't be easy," he said thoughtfully. "Maybe I was meant to see the lives I changed. What if I took life without exchanging it for lessons that would have made me a better person?"

"Do you think you might have killed people and that's what the dreams are about?" I asked.

"I'm sure people died from what I did," he said. "There were probably even some civilians, but not children. What would children be doing on boats?"

His words startled me and I wasn't sure I had heard him correctly. "Boats?" I asked. "Just what did you do over there?"

"We were assigned to interrupt transportation and shipping but there weren't many bridges or rail lines that hadn't already been destroyed. Mostly we went after shipping, usually in the Rhine and its tributaries."

For the second time that afternoon, I sat stunned by the extraordinary that lived within a story. If Jeff noticed the surprise in my eyes or the slight tremble of my hand, he didn't say anything. Most likely, he thought I was simply lost in thought over the puzzle that he had brought to me. I encouraged Jeff to give his troubled nights a little more time, that perhaps he was confronting issues that he hadn't yet resolved in his life, issues that he may not even be aware of.

"The body has a miraculous way of healing," I told Jeff, "even when we don't realize that we need it. Why don't we let things go as they are for a while before we get in the way and throw medications at the problem."

Healing was well underway when I paused in surprise at the door to the waiting room a short time later. Like Heidi, Jeff sat there waiting for a ride from a family member. They sat next to each other engaged in conversation, punctuated with broad smiles and laughter. They could have been old friends.

I wish I had paid closer attention in physics class. Perhaps theories of relativity, non-linear time, and time as a spatial dimension would have helped explain what I was seeing, but it wouldn't make it less miraculous. It wasn't important that I understood, only that I was aware of the power of time and synchronicity. I had often wondered why a German-born lady would find herself in the Appalachian countryside and why a corporate executive would choose to live out the last of his life in this place. The answer now seems as simple as it is obvious: it is the unfolding of the universe.

I would not speak to Heidi or Jeff about each other. Although blessed by it, it was not my story to share. In time they would figure it out, of that I was certain. I stood in that doorway for the longest time thrilled by the happiness I saw in their faces. It was as if they had met as mere children so very long ago, but of course, it was only a moment ago.

CHAPTER 13

I'm so Happy

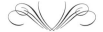

Friendship is a single soul dwelling in two bodies.

ARISTOTLE

*The nearer people approach old age the closer they
return to a semblance of childhood.*

DESIDERIUS ERASMUS

While most physicians are oblivious to it, there is much fear
and pain in medicine. When I start my day in the office, there
is almost always a patient in the waiting room with pain. A pulled
back, a twisted knee, an ache in the belly—the ways in which a person
can hurt is seemingly endless. So too sits a patient with fear—afraid
of an expected treatment, apprehension over lost control, or fear of
what might be found in the examination room down the hall. Some
diagnoses are feared more than others.

Hardly a week goes by that I do not encounter the fear of cancer.
Some have the disease and meet every laboratory test, scan, and
follow-up visit with apprehension. Most, however, fear that a both-
ersome symptom—fatigue, an ache, or even a lump on the skin—is

certain to be cancer. Everyone it seems knows someone with cancer. Everyone knows a horror story about invasive diagnostic procedures or cures that are worse than the disease. A family member, a good friend, or the boss at work—everyone knows someone who has died from cancer and they sit in the waiting room in fear.

If few words strike greater fear in the hearts of people than cancer, dementia is certainly one of them. Forgotten car keys, difficulty remembering names, and even errors balancing the checkbook are enough to drive older patients to their doctors. They are terrified.

"I went to the garage this morning," a middle-aged man recently told me, "and when I got there I had forgotten what it was I was going to do. It's the second time this week. It's how the guy started down the street. He has it so bad he can't feed himself. I just know that I've got it too."

Few diseases I have encountered in medicine have a greater reach than dementia. It inflicts families, marriages, and friendships as nobody suffer its effects alone. In fact, those with the disease may actually have an easier time than those around them. There is seldom pain and the fear of expectations gradually surrenders to failing memory and confusion. For caretakers and those who are left to watch, it can be a difficult and terrifying journey.

Dementia is not a stranger on the medicine floors at the Teaching Hospital. It is among the most prevalent diagnoses of nursing home patients and when nursing home patients become ill, they invariably find their way to the Teaching Hospital. With them come long medication lists, antibiotic-resistant infections, and families in pain.

I stopped by the medicine floor one evening to check up on a patient before heading home. She had had a blood clot to her lung and needed to stay in the hospital until she was on the proper dose of blood thinners. She looked great and I was surprised that she didn't complain about not going home that day. While she never would have admitted it, I believe she was fascinated by the admission of Maddie Holcomb to the bed next to hers earlier in the day. Maddie had Alzheimer's disease and the spectacle of harried residents caring for her, the dynamics of family that stood by her bed, and the seeming ravings of an old woman was better than watching reality television at home.

As I wrote my progress note in the nursing station, I took interest in the young doctor that was taking care of Maddie; indeed, he looked harried and the night was still young. Like most of my colleagues, I looked back on my own internship with nostalgia and the longing for those simpler days. It is amazing how time can heal and change our perspective of events. As I watched, I could see myself sitting in his place. Internship seemed only a moment ago and gone was the nostalgia. While there were good days, there were also dark ones.

It was the dark days of internship that gave me the most. Sleepless nights spent caring for the sickest of the sick honed skills that will bless me forever. Holding a patient's hand when the medications weren't enough nourished contemplation that perhaps curing was not enough. And when long days merged into long weeks and the pain of others seemed unendurable, there was extraordinary friendship.

I would always sit next to Ryan Charles during morning report when we were interns. Sometimes I bought the coffee, other times he did. It was the conference when interns would present patients that they had admitted to the chief resident and the program director. It was always a stressful hour and a culmination of stressful nights spent with patients ill beyond belief.

Of all the admissions that could come a medicine intern's way at the Teaching Hospital, by far the most dreaded was the nursing home transfer. It always meant sick patients, long hours, and hard work that seldom made a difference. It was not a rare occurrence; in fact, it became strangely predictable—weekends, holidays, and night shifts at the nursing home. So too was the reason that most patients were transferred—*altered mental status.*

"Altered mental status," I heard Ryan say one morning in frustration. "It's the third one this week and not one of them could talk or get out of bed at baseline. How in the world do they know that their mental status has changed?"

It was never hard, however, to find a problem in a nursing home patient to justify the hospital admission. So we set about treating urinary tract infections, dehydration, and bedsores before sending them back to the nursing home. Sometimes it would take a month or two before the nursing home would send the patient back to us— sometimes it was mere hours—and the process would start anew.

Perhaps it was the battlefield camaraderie of internship, maybe it was the long and stressful hours, or it might have been the coffee, but Ryan and I became friends. It was a friendship unlike any other I had known. It was as if the harshness of our surroundings had cracked the shells that we spent a lifetime building and through the exposed crevice, we could see deep into each other's soul. I liked what I saw.

If our friendship was forged in the heat of internship, it would grow exponentially when we would slip beyond the bounds of diagnosis and cure. It is amazing how quickly one forgets the power of family and the fulfillment of companionship when away from home in a strange city and challenged by work. Perhaps it is the first step of life being consumed by work and ultimately work becoming one's life. If that was to have been my fate, Ryan would have none of it.

What started as lunch away from work, an occasional movie, or even a game of golf gradually became dinner at his home or an afternoon spent with his family. It didn't take long—before I even knew what was happening—for me to become part of his family. I watched his family grow and shared in their joys and sorrows. I was a part of every family gathering. As I sat watching his children open their presents one Christmas morning, I worried that I might be experiencing life vicariously through the grace of others. Now, many miles farther along on my journey, I recognize the importance of savoring life any way possible, if not through direct experience then through the lives of others. It was, and is, a precious gift.

Dinner at Ed and Libby Charles's home was part of that gift. Ryan's parents were a few years older than my own, but every time I was with them, I could feel the love and wisdom that had filled my childhood. If I couldn't be home on special days, there was no place I would have rather been than with his parents.

Libby amazed me. After raising eleven children, she returned to school to become an English professor. Her dinners were always served with rich stories from literature, wonders of travel, and the joy she found in her family. More than once Ryan would sit red-faced at the dinner table as his mother would thrill her guests with a story from his youth that he would have rather not shared. Libby was a bit forgetful in those days and always joined in the laughter when the meal's roast had been placed in the freezer instead of the oven, coffee was brewed without the grounds, and dessert was served before the entrée. We didn't know it then, but there were dark clouds on the horizon.

I was a mass of conflicted emotion—flattered to exhilaration and intimidated to the point of nausea when Ed and Libby Charles first appeared in my office as patients. I had long felt uncomfortable having friends as patients, but Ed and Libby were more than friends. It would be like taking care of my parents, but I could not say no to them. As time passed, it became clear that Libby's forgetfulness was more than something to laugh about at the dinner table.

I saw all the clues. She had trouble with numbers and seemed to struggle with words that an English teacher would know. She would fake her way through conversations with old friends that she had forgotten. She never left her husband's side. I saw all the clues and they made me sick. Libby had Alzheimer's disease.

I had watched the relentless march of Alzheimer's many times before, but it was always through the eyes of the physician. This was different. This was personal. Libby was family. I watched powerless as her confusion grew. I grieved for the sharp mind of the teacher that was lost somewhere in vast emptiness we call dementia. I mourned her loss of story. Perhaps being a physician made it all the worse as I knew what awaited her around the bend of the road ahead.

As more and more of the Libby that her family knew disappeared, they struggled to fill the void that they felt in their lives, but it could not be done. It couldn't even be understood. When she became disoriented and started to wander, she required constant attention. Occasionally, she had become lost on their apartment building floor. There was no more devoted a husband than Ed. Though he tried, his eyes could not remain open all the time and he could not will away the need for sleep. There were tears in Ed's eyes the day he asked me to help watch over Libby at the nursing home he had reluctantly selected for her. While his children had urged the move for some time, he couldn't help but feel he had failed the person he most loved.

Libby was not alone in her plight. The number of patients with dementia at the nursing home shocked me on my first visit there. The dayrooms were filled with graying heads and faces that begged to tell a story. Some sat expressionless in wheelchairs lost in thought or the unknown. Most sat at tables with childlike delight at games and crafts placed before them. A few wandered about exuding a curiosity about every corner or what might be seen through every window.

Libby was one of the wanderers. She would walk endlessly about her small world protected by door alarms, secured cabinets, and watchful eyes. She carried a baby doll wherever she went. Occasionally, she would stop and sit to attend to its needs. It seemed strangely appropriate that she had returned to a time when she was most happy: caring for children.

Libby was well cared for at the nursing home. I marveled at the staff's patience and gentle ways with souls that marched to the sound of a drummer that only they could hear. Libby's every need was met and if the staff could not provide the love that she once knew, she did not want for it. Ed brought it with him every day. He would sit with her for hours and when she wanted to wander, he would tag along with her and experience joy in her every discovery. It was the happiest I had seen Ed in years. Still, there was sadness behind his smile and guilt that he could not provide for his wife at home.

There was little I could do for Libby on my visits. I would listen to her heart and lungs, review the nursing notes, and sign the inevitable paperwork that had accumulated since my last tip. Mostly I would just sit with her, wishing I could do more.

Libby had ventured far down dementia's dark path when I stopped to see her one afternoon during my lunch break. There was a time when I would always start my visit by searching for where her wandering had taken her, but it had been many months since she had left her bed unassisted. On this day though, her room sat empty. The nursing staff's confusion led to concern when a search of the usual places that a resident might have been taken in a wheelchair did not locate her. Libby had grown increasingly frail and she was requiring greater assistance with even simple tasks. It seemed unlikely that she would have left her room alone.

We found her in a patient's room at the end of a back corridor; it was the last room to be searched. Next to the elderly man's bed, Libby sat in a chair gently rocking the baby doll she held in her arms. The nurse told me that the old man had fallen recently and fractured his hip and was not doing well. Libby grinned like that of a child who had been discovered in a forbidden place. Clutching her baby doll and with an occasional giggle, Libby walked slowly back to her room with me.

I sat in Libby's room and read through her chart. As she required more personal attention, the number and length of progress notes increased. Lost in the words, I was startled by a voice. "How's your mother doing, Bill?"

I glanced about the room expectantly but Libby and I were alone. She was sitting on the side of her bed watching me. Her eyes seemed different. There was a focus in her gaze that I had not seen since the days we used to laugh while gathered around the dinner table. There was enormous warmth in her smile.

"How's you mother doing, Bill?" she asked.

While it was not unusual for those with dementia to have lucid periods, I had never encountered it so vividly. She had not recognized me for well over a year, and then only as someone vaguely familiar.

"She's doing well, Libby," I replied with a slight stutter in my voice.

"You need to call her more often," she gently scolded.

"I'll call her tonight," I said softly.

"Has Ed been in for a check-up?" she asked. "He looks so tired and takes care of everyone but himself."

"He's doing fine, Libby," I reassured her. "I'll make sure he comes in soon."

"Have you seen Ryan recently?" she asked.

"Just last week," I replied. "We had lunch together. He's doing fine too, Libby."

"I love them so," she said wistfully.

"They know, Libby," I said with a catch in my voice, "and they love you."

She sat quiet for several moments fidgeting with a button on her nightgown and then looked at me a bit quizzically, almost as if she didn't know who I was. The focus was gone from her eyes—replaced by an almost magical innocence. With a trembling hand, she reached for the baby doll sitting on her nightstand and brought it close to her chest.

Climbing into bed, she rolled onto her side and cuddled her baby doll. "I'm so happy," she said to me with a childlike grin before closing her eyes and drifting off to sleep. It would be the last time I would see Libby, but her journey had left an indelible presence in my life that would guide me on my own travels. It was wisdom that might have eluded me had it not been for those dark days of internship.

Loud voices brought my attention back to the present moment. Maddie Holcomb's daughter was arguing with the intern caring for her mother.

"What do you mean she's going back to the nursing home tomorrow?" the woman asked incredulously.

"Ma'am," the young doctor said patiently, "she was admitted

slightly dehydrated. It could have been corrected in the emergency room but we kept her overnight. She's had IV fluids and is back to her baseline. She doesn't need to be in the hospital any longer.

"Back to her baseline?" the angry woman shouted. "My mother won a Pulitzer Prize in journalism. Does that look like that woman down the hall? She's wearing diapers for heaven's sake. We can't have people seeing her like this. She's like a little baby in there. She's worse than when we first put her in the home."

"She has Alzheimer's, ma'am," the exasperated doctor said. "I can't fix that, nobody can. All we can do is correct the acute problem. Sometimes it's hard to get patients with this problem to drink enough water and they become dehydrated. That we can fix—and we have—but your mother still has Alzheimer's. When was the last time you saw her?"

"It's been awhile," the daughter said, clearly taken aback by the question.

"Alzheimer's is progressive," the doctor explained, "and sometimes things deteriorate more quickly than other times. It sounds like she lost some function between the time you saw her last and now. I realize it's not much consolation, but she appears to be getting excellent care."

Indeed, it was little consolation, whether for the children of a journalist, the husband of a teacher, or the brother of a farmer. Alzheimer's was the ultimate equalizer. It didn't matter the occupation, the size of the bank account, or the amount of education; the journey they walked was eerily similar.

After I finished my paperwork, I stopped by my patient's room one last time before heading off to home. The nurse was busy checking the IV and the welfare of her patient so I stood off to the side and waited until she was finished. I felt uncomfortably conspicuous standing close to Maddie Holcomb's bed as I waited, but I was fascinated watching a sliver of her life unfold. Her daughter sat next to her bed with red eyes and a face streaked with tears born from her mother's pain. Perhaps I had grown numb to it through the years, but as I studied Maddie, I could not see the pain.

Despite snow-white hair, wrinkled skin, and a hint of frailty, Maddie reminded me of a child. She seemed oblivious to the worry that swirled around her as she toyed with the snack that had been placed on her bedside table. I felt her excitement and childlike awe in everything around her, but I could not feel pain. Perhaps her journey had taken her back to the way it was before; before she knew such things as desire, need, and achievement. Maybe it's the journey that we are all on; to once again experience the innocence of childhood before we learned the expectations of others. We come into this world free of concern, wanting nothing, and delighting in the experience of being. There is something comforting in the possibility that we might leave the world as we first found it. It is a place where there is no pain. The pain is for those of us left behind who do not yet understand.

I smiled at Maddie as she looked up at me. There was a twinkle in her eye; the same twinkle I had seen at Ryan's home as his children opened their presents on Christmas morning. With a delighted squeal, Maddie inserted a finger deep into the cup of chocolate ice cream that sat in front of her. A grin that stretched from ear to ear grew across her face as she looked into my eyes.

"I'm so happy," she said.

While not everyone around her could see it, I knew beyond all doubt that Maddie's journey was unfolding as it should; just as Libby's had. Perhaps the journey is not as dark as we had feared.

CHAPTER 14

The Uncertain Gift

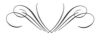

*Do you not see how necessary a world of pain and troubles
is to school an intelligence and make it a soul?*

JOHN KEATS

*Clouds come floating into my life, no longer to carry rain
or usher storm, but to add color to my sunset sky.*

RABINDRANATH TAGORE

I searched my memory for a time when the telephone rang in the middle of the night with good news or to bring calm to my life, but I couldn't recall such an event. At times I had even wondered why we had such devices installed in our homes. I glanced at the clock beside my bed as the phone rang for the second time. It was 2:02 am. Oddly, I almost welcomed the interruption of the night that had brought no sleep and peace that I was unable to feel through its quiet.

Although it was a little raspy, I instantly recognized the voice on the phone as that of Wilbur Morton. He was a nice man, but he was quite a worrier. He worked as a used car salesman but his expertise was in the world of the *what if*. He was just in the office the week before to review the results of blood work that I had ordered. It wasn't really time for his routine lab tests but I ordered them early hoping to bring some peace to a life that thought way too much of disease and illness. After spending ten minutes explaining the meaning of every laboratory study printed on the report, all of which were well within the normal range, I asked him why he looked so concerned.

"What if," he replied nervously, "the laboratory made a mistake and the tests aren't normal? How will we know if I'm sick?"

With a deep breath, I laid in the darkness and asked Mr. Morton what I could do for him.

"Doc," he croaked into the phone, "I think I need to go the hospital. I'm sure I have stripped throat."

It took some effort to stifle a laugh, but it was not lost on me that it was the first smile that crossed my face in well over a day and I felt strangely appreciative. I couldn't help but wonder what a stripped throat would look like. Perhaps it was one not wearing any clothes.

"Why would you go to the hospital for that, Mr. Morton?" I asked in the most serious-sounding voice I could muster.

"I know you could call antibiotics in to the pharmacy for me," he explained, "but they can give it to you directly into the veins at the hospital. It will work faster."

If it wasn't so frustrating, my patients' pursuit of antibiotics would have fascinated me. Where in the crossroads of history did the belief emerge that every cold, every cough, and every fever could be immediately eradicated with antibiotics? It was a conversation that I had many times every week in the office—that colds are caused by viruses that antibiotics cannot treat, the risk of antibiotic resistance, and that the body's immune system will quickly speed them to recovery—only to have the same conversation the following week. However, I had never had the conversation in the middle of the night.

I suspect that the belief that doctors had a pill for every ailment is a monster of our own making, however. It is so much easier to write a prescription than it is to explain to a dubious patient why an antibiotic is not the best for them. It can take a half-hour to calm an anxious soul when a tranquilizer can be written in seconds. Pain pills quickly ease the back pain—and make the exam room available for the next patient—while discussing exercise and altered lifestyles takes longer. And prescribing antidepressants? Well, it can be mercifully less painful than listening to the story.

Mr. Morton seemed reassured by our discussion and eager to try salt-water gargles and throat lozenges for a while. He was about to hang up when almost as an afterthought he thought he asked, "You don't think this could be throat cancer, do you?"

"Certainly not," I said, obviously confused. "You've had this for just a few hours. Why would you think about throat cancer?"

An embarrassed-sounding voice replied, "Well, that's what dad died from."

"If I recall correctly," I said, "dad was a heavy smoker, he chewed tobacco, and he drank. You don't do any of those things. But you know something, Wilbur, there is energy in what we think about, just like there is energy in illness. Maybe healing is nothing more than restoring our body's energy to levels that sustain and nurture us. What we spend our day thinking about can make us feel bad. Have you ever felt yourself sick with worry? The good news is that your thoughts can also make you feel good. Try to spend a few minutes every day doing something that makes you feel good—reading an inspirational book, listening to music, or taking a walk—and I'm willing to bet you will find yourself feeling better."

The clock read 2:31 am when I hung up that phone and I had yet to sleep that night. Perhaps Wilbur's call was not just an opportunity to share lessons that my teachers left with me long ago, but a chance to be touched by their wisdom once again myself. It is truly amazing how they find a way to come to me when I need them the most. My thoughts had indeed been troubled, and while that was not an uncommon happening at the end of a week spent immersed deep in the currents of medicine, the waters seemed uncommonly dark. Sleep or not, in the morning I would head for the shelter of my woods. There was much healing to be done.

My teachers made the drive with me; many had not visited my thoughts for many years. David Trasket was there. I hadn't felt the burning of smoke in my throat for decades but his council of trusting what you feel in your heart and assurances that we are never alone were whispered in my soul only a moment ago. Even he would have found irony in his lessons of firefighting that had found their way into the making of a physician. He was right. There comes a time when we discover that what we know and that which we have been taught are not enough. We discover there is something more, even though we probably do not understand what that more might be. It was in the discovery that healing became possible.

It was at the VA hospital that Byron Weeks found that great order and meaning hides within chaos. Of the many potent medicines and treatments he ordered there, the young doctor discovered that the giving of himself through listening and touch was his most powerful tool. In those same halls, Thomas Shipe discovered that listening could unlock the wisdom that is woven within one's story. He had contemplated a religious life, but instead was drawn to serve in a different way. As Byron and Thomas listened, they discovered healing and became my teachers.

Driving along those seldom traveled gravel roads that would eventually lead me to Demazie Hollow, I was not oblivious to the fact that some of my greatest teachers came from the wooded hills and color-soaked meadows that I now passed. They didn't have advanced degrees—some couldn't read or even write their name—but they were master teachers. Some found their way to the clinic to share their lessons. Others I would pass on a wooded trail or happen across while lingering along the banks of a crystal clear stream. Sometimes they would seek me out while standing in a line at a gas station.

They were teachers that knew about scarcity and abundance and how each is but a thought away. Some had been victims and only by giving up their past and seizing the present moment could they teach about healing. Many were oblivious of the poverty from which they came and through giving of what little they had discovered lives filled with incredible richness. Some were students of nature and of the energy that ebbs and flows across the ridges and through the valleys. It is the same energy that lives within our thoughts—energy that can make us ill or lead us to healing—that empowers us to change how we feel in an instant. Some demonstrated that whatever we might need in this life is ours to attract—it's but a thought away.

Betts Unger was waiting for me at Demazie Hollow. She was always there. I heard her voice in every bird's song and could feel her presence in my every step. She taught me how to find wonder everywhere I might look; you find it by looking for it and by expecting to find it. She helped me discover the wisdom that can be found in nature; wisdom that flows from the immensity of the universe and that links us to everything that has ever been and everything that will ever be. Medical school taught me all about diagnosis and cure, but it wasn't until I could look upon my patients with wonder and appreciate the wisdom that was woven within their souls that healing became possible.

Only the arrogance that is possible in a physician could foster the belief that healing is a need reserved solely for patients. Sometimes we need it the most. Perhaps it was those early teachers that rode with me in the back of an ambulance or called out from a crowd that had gathered to witness a spectacular automobile accident, but I have been deeply touched by the brevity and uncertainty of life. Life can change in the blink of an eye. It is an awareness that can stifle our days with worry or enrich them with moments lived most thoroughly.

Medicine can be a risky business. Venture too close to the lives of your patients and you can feel their pain, become friends, and risk sleepless nights worrying about them, and should they become family, your life may never be the same. Still, if healing is to be found, it will be in the closeness, the friendship, and in family.

"Why do bad things have to happen?" the young doctor had asked me just the morning before at the Teaching Hospital. He struggled to hide his humanity—moist eyes, a quiver of the lip, and a catch in his voice—as he had worked hard to become a professional. It seemed a plaintive plea from the wilderness and it begged for understanding. Few words have ever touched me so deeply.

Sitting on that ancient rock beneath the great red oak in Demazie Hollow, the pain of that young doctor's words gradually eased their icy grip on my soul. The morning mist still lingered just above the treetops and cast a mystical glow across autumn's spectacular show. It was hard to imagine pain and darkness in this place, although more than once the thought of fire and what it could do to the hollow brought me worry. I felt Betts and the wisdom she helped me find in the natural world with particular keenness at those times. Perhaps it is in our perceptions and expectations—and not reality—that things are bad. As horrible as fire might first seem to be to the forest, once the smoke clears it can be seen as a gift, albeit an uncertain one, that becomes essential to its continued growth and health. Maybe it is that way with our journey as well.

While Jerry Ritchie and Rachel were companions for many years, they did not discover love until Jerry discovered illness. It was in that discovery that they grasped the present moment and lived a fullness beyond comprehension. And while those that observed believed their love to be all too brief, love in the present moment lasted a lifetime. It could have been a journey absent the sweetness of love, but dying saved their lives.

Through the horrors of illness and that which modern medicine can impose upon the soul, Jacob Keller lost memories of the past and the desire to dream of the future. He lived in the only place left to him—the present moment—and he took his wife Janice on the journey with him. Together they experienced a gift that few will ever come to know—the chance to fall in love a second time and to live in a paradise free of past regrets. In that paradise, perhaps too short for some, they lived a lifetime.

Libby Ryan lived in darkness that so many of us fear. While she felt no pain, those around her lived the horror of her forgotten accomplishments, her lost intellect, and her childlike state. Without her memories, Libby was sentenced to live out her life in the present moment. It was there that she was able to conclude her journey in happiness.

Like the jack pines of Northern Michigan that cannot seed the forest floor until their cones are touched by flame, so too are our journeys made complete by the seeming adversity of life. It is a gift made possible through the universal intelligence of synchronicity, non-linear time, and a connection with all things. Perhaps the greatest gift, however, is for those that watch the journey and are left behind.

It was that way with Juanita's yet-to-be doctor in a sweltering Texas hospital. While they did not understand each other's words, she taught him how to speak with caring presence and quiet. Through her illness that he could not cure, he discovered healing. A part of Juanita travels with him on his own journey and blesses all that might call him doctor.

It was that way as well with that young doctor at the Teaching Hospital.

Mitchell Breuer was one of our senior residents and while it was still early in the training year, his ward team functioned with machinelike precision. He ran his team with the wisdom gleaned from the Cold War arms treaties; *trust but verify.* It was so much easier to do all the work himself and he probably could have taken care of all twelve patients on his service without anyone's help, but that is not how young doctors learned at the Teaching Hospital. He missed the security he felt as an intern when he knew every minute detail about his patients. Now all he knew about his patients was what he was told or sly enough to figure out for himself.

Mitchell gave the interns who worked under him a great deal of autonomy. After all, others had done it for him and the responsibility had taught him much. He asked only that his interns check in with him every two hours. While he tried hard to stay out of their way, he quietly monitored their progress by following every laboratory result from a computer in one of the nursing units.

It had been a busy day for admissions and Mitchell lost track of time. Sitting at a computer, he scrolled through his patients' reports while he paged each of his team members to check on their progress. The medical students promptly answered his pages as being on their own too long made them crazy. His interns were a different story, and that made Mitchell crazy. Thirty minutes and four pages later, he couldn't take watching a silent telephone any longer and he set out looking for the rest of his team.

"Hey, Dr. Foster," he shouted across a nursing station at one of his interns, "don't you answer pages any more?"

His intern jumped in response and sheepishly noted that the display on his pager had grown dark. "Sorry," he mumbled.

"How many times have I told you guys to change the battery in your pagers every morning?" Mitchell asked without expecting an answer. "What if there had been a code?"

He sat down with his young charge, who wasn't that much younger than himself, and reviewed the orders he had written on his new patient. He couldn't help but feel pride in the work. The patient was severely dehydrated and the fluid-replacement calculations could be challenging for interns. He couldn't have done better himself, he beamed in delight.

"Now," he said while trying to paint a stern look on his face, "Have you seen your partner in crime?"

"Not since lunch," the intern replied.

"Fine," Mitchell grumbled. "I guess I'm going on a hunt, but when I get back we are all taking a field trip down to the telephone operators and learn how to change the batteries in our pagers."

And hunt he did. He checked the emergency room, the cafeteria, and the residents' lounge. Floor by floor, he checked every nursing station and asked every ward clerk, but nobody had seen his intern.

More bewildered than angry, he checked the hospital lobby, the gift shop and even the bank of vending machines by the elevators, but to no avail.

"There had better not be anyone in here," he thought to himself with a touch of anger as he turned the key in the lock of the residents' call room. But there was someone there. His intern lay motionless across the floor.

The reflexes of his training kicked in. He checked for a pulse. There was none. He checked for breathing. There was none. The reflexes of his humanity kicked in. They were not as polished and hadn't been used in some time, but they filled his eyes with tears as he contemplated what he was about to do—resuscitate a colleague; a friend.

He delivered breaths. He delivered chest compressions—so many compressions. Many minutes passed and he knew he was in trouble. Nobody would ever find them in the little used call rooms. He pulled the telephone from the desk by its cord and waited in desperation for the operator to answer. He delivered breaths. He delivered chest compressions, so many chest compressions before the sounds of panicked voices and the rumbling of a crash cart could be heard approaching a part of the hospital where they had never ventured before.

A tube was placed into the trachea and with the squeeze of a bag, oxygen was forced into the young physician's lungs. An intravenous catheter was inserted into a vein in the neck. Monitoring electrodes were attached to the chest. It was a well-rehearsed dance and the performance seemed more urgent than most.

Defibrillator paddles were placed to the chest and shocks of energy delivered with a jolt that made everyone jump. Chest compressions were delivered. Rounds of chemicals were pushed into the veins followed by even more powerful shocks of electricity. Still more compressions, more chemicals, and even more shocks.

Tears streaming down his face, Mitchell looked at his watch. They had been there an hour. Every pair of eyes but one focused intently on the senior resident. "Time of death," he managed to say, but not another word was possible. He sat in shocked disbelief.

Sam was dead.

Twenty-six years old, a newlywed, and a physician for mere months and she was gone.

"Why do bad things have to happen?" Sam's colleague had asked me the morning before. They had started internship together. It was a question that seemed to have no answer, but of course, there was an answer.

"If I should die tomorrow," I remember her saying once, "I shall do so knowing that I have lived my dream." It is something that few of us can say, not because our lives have lacked abundance or completeness, but because we have been unable to see that which happens now and appreciate the moment. Living a dream does not rest in yesterday's accomplishments or tomorrow's hope. It lives in the awareness of today and in the happiness that can be found only in the here and now.

Sam discovered in mere months what many physicians spend long careers looking for but never finding in medicine. The ability to cure disease, ease symptoms, and prolong life is simply not enough. The meaning lies in healing. It requires skills not taught in medical school or discussed in journals. It requires a willingness to consider possibilities greater than ourselves and even our understanding. Sometimes it requires a gentle touch, a listening ear, or perhaps a tear-filled eye. Sam understood it is in helping others heal that our lives are healed as well.

Sam's colleagues will be forever changed by the brief time she walked among them. They will never look at patients quite the same way because of Sam. Some will hear stories that they never listened for before. Some will see miracles that they had never before thought possible. Some will become healers. That, of course, was the answer her young colleague had struggled for and whose pain had touched my heart. He didn't realize it yet but Sam had been his teacher, as she had been mine.

The whistle of the tufted titmouse drew my gaze upward into the canopy of the red oak. As if on cue, it floated downward like a leaf to come to a clinging stop on a rhododendron that grew nearby. Its gray crest rose and fell with every excited chirp as if acknowledging my presence in what was its special place as well. I felt Betts sitting on that rock with me, thrilling in the wonders I had learned to see.

A spicebush swallowtail drifted by on an invisible cushion of air. It was Jack Hoff's favorite butterfly and I knew that he too was nearby. He shared a wisdom that was as timeless as the rock upon which I sat. Through his extraordinary stories that I did not understand at the time, I came to see the extraordinary in my patients' eyes. They too had their stories—wisdom that bubbled up from the depths of their souls—and in them I found secrets that make healing possible.

We came into this world—it was only a moment ago—filled with endless happiness, unbounded peace, and seeds carried from another place that have the potential to grow into incredible aware-ness. We learned our lessons well and as the expectations, fears, and attitudes of others became our own, we forgot the gifts that we came here with. Perhaps healing is the journey that we take to once again find that peace. It is a journey with many twists and turns but there are many teachers along the way to keep us centered upon our path. The journey is far too brief—it takes a lifetime.